# LESIONS of the JAW BONE:
## RADIOGRAPHIC FEATURES

# LESIONS of the JAW BONE:
## RADIOGRAPHIC FEATURES

*By*

**VIVIAN J. HARRIS, M.D.**
*Chairman, Department of Radiology*
*Cook County Hospital*
*Professor, Department of Radiology*
*University of Illinois*

**FELIX R. LAWRENCE, D.D.S.**
*Chairman, Division of Dentistry and*
*Section of Oral and Maxillofacial Surgery*
*Cook County Hospital*

**JUSTO RODRIGUEZ, M.D.**
*Chief, Section of Otolaryngology and*
*Tomography*
*Cook County Hospital*
*Assistant Professor*
*Chicago Medical School*

**WARREN H. GREEN, INC.**
*St. Louis, Missouri, U.S.A.*

*Published by*

WARREN H. GREEN, INC.
8356 Olive Boulevard
St. Louis, Missouri 63132, U.S.A.

ISBN Number 87527-212-6

*Printed in the United States of America*

# PREFACE

We have attempted to demonstrate various tumor masses and disorders of the jawbones, both common and rare, selected from the large number of cases available to us in Cook County Hospital. Although our emphasis has been on masses which occur in children, diseases of adults are also included.

While reviewing much of our material we were struck with the similarity of the radiographic appearance of many disorders. This finding impressed upon us the fact that the final diagnosis in many instances can only be made when clinical features and histopathology are known.

While these tumors are presented from conventional radiography some of the newer modalities in imaging such as CAT scanning and Nuclear Imaging may, on occasion, help to confirm a diagnosis or outline the limits of a tumor. A few examples are included in this volume.

We are grateful to many persons who assisted in the preparation of this book. Many physicians contributed generously with radiographic and histopathologic sections. We are grateful to Dr. Paul Szanto of the Department of Pathology, Cook County Hospital for his assistance with the pathology and to Dr. Harvey White, Dr. G. Espinoza and Dr. W.P. Cockshott for radiographs they contributed and Dr. J. Seibert for a clinical photograph. We would like to express our appreciation to Miss Deborah Wilson who patiently typed the manuscript; we are indebted to Ms. Cheryl Haugh who prepared the schematic drawings and assisted with much of the photography.

# CONTENTS

# LESIONS of the JAW BONE:
## RADIOGRAPHIC FEATURES

# 1

## THE PANORAMIC EXAMINATION OF THE MANDIBLE

### PANTOMOGRAPHY

Pantomography is a special radiographic technique which produces a panoramic roentogenogram. The examination is based on the principle of body section radiography. During this procedure, the x-ray tube and the film both rotate while the patient remains stationary. As a result, a radiograph of the mandible is obtained which includes the entire mandible, both temporo-mandibular joints, maxilla and the teeth in the same planes.

There is a minimal distortion and superimposition of shadows; the relationship of the teeth to each other and the jaw is well demonstrated. Magnification, as in geometrical tomography, can be used for better delineation and demonstration of the osseous structures.

Although panoramic radiography has been used in dentistry and oral surgery as a screening procedure, the oral surgeon who is dealing with large lesions derives maximum benefits from this procedure since he obtains an entire survey of the maxillo-facial structures. For this reason, panoramic radiography is of vital importance in the diagnosis and treatment of the patient with maxillo-facial pathology.

Different panoramic units using the same tomographic principle have been used in the United States such as Panorex (S.S. White Co.), Orthopanto-mography (Seimen's Co.), G.E. 3000 (General Electric Co.).

In Cook County Hospital, with an average of 6,000 panoramic examinations per year, panoramic x-ray has been used in the evaluation and follow-ups of the following pathological conditions:

1. Trauma — Fractures of the maxillary sinus and orbit
   a. Trimalleolar fracture.
   b. Isolated fracture of the orbit.
   c. Fracture of the body and ramus of the mandible.
   d. Fracture of the coronoid process of the mandible and fracture of the condyle.
   e. Fracture of the zygomatic arch.

f. LeFort I, II and III.
2. Congenital anomalies of the mandible.
3. Radiographic manifestations of systemic disease.
   a. Paget's disease.
   b. Osteogenesis imperfecta, osteopetrosis.
   c. Pseudohypoparathyroidism, hyperparathyroidism.
4. Benign and malignant lesions of the jaw.
5. Location of supernumerality.
6. Pre and post operative patients.

The time needed for the procedure, the low cost and the lower radiation are advantages compared with the conventional x-ray. This procedure often is performed as a supplement to the intra-oral examination and the conventional x-ray.

In the past, panoramic radiography has been used in otolarynogology radiology in the early detection of carcinoma of the maxillary sinus and other malignant lesions of the oral cavity. It has been used also in the diagnosis of benign lesions of the maxillary sinus like mucous retention cysts, osteomas and mucocele. Despite the new advances in computer tomography, panoramic examination of the mandible remains one of the best tools for diagnosis and treatment of the patient with maxillo-facial conditions.

## References

1. Brueggemann, A.: Evaluation of the Panorex Unit. Oral Surg., 24:348-358, 1967.
2. Jacobson, A.F., and Ferguson, J.P.: Evaluation of the S.S. White Panorex X-ray Machine. Pub. No. (FDA) 72-8020, BRH-DEP 72-6, Department of Health, Education and Welfare, U.S. Government Print Office.
3. Manson-Hing, L.R.: Advances in Dental Pantomography: The GE 3000 Oral Surg., 31:430-438, 1971.
4. Manson-Hing, L.R.: Evaluation of Radiographic Techniques, Including Pantomography. J. Am. Dent. Assoc., 87:145-154, 1973.
5. Manson-Hing, L.R.: Pantomography Today. Oral Surg., 34:832-837, 1971.
6. McMahon, J.J.: Head and Neck Exposures from Panoramix Roentgenography. Oral Surg., 31:122-132, 1970.
7. Schaffer, A.W.: The Panoramix in Oral Surgery. Oral Surg., 24:359-363, 1967.
8. Schramek, J.M., et al.: Panoramic Radiography in Head and Neck Pathology. Laryngoscope, 80:1797-1808, 1970.

9. Schramek, J.M., and Rappaport, I.: Panoramic X-ray Screening for Early Detection of Maxillary Sinus Malignancy. Arch Otolaryngol, 90:347-351, 1969.
10. Smith, C.J., and Fleming, R.D.: A Comprehensive Review of Normal Anatomic Landmarks and Artifacts as Visualized on Panorex Radiology. Oral Surg., 34:291-304, 1974.
11. Updegrave, W.J.: Visualizing the Mandibular Ramus in Panoramic Radiography. Oral Surg., 31:422-479, 1971.

# 2

# CYSTS OF THE JAWS

## BENIGN CYSTS

Benign cysts of the jaw are common and may originate from various sources (1-3) which may be those associated with tooth elements or arise from proliferation of Hertwig's sheath due to pulp inflammations. Embryonal inclusions may give rise to cysts. Cysts may also occur secondary to trauma. The pathogenesis of cyst formation is thought to start with the breakdown of a group of proliferated epithelial cells, the central cells necrosing because of poor blood supply, thereby initiating cavitation. Protein which breaks down from the degenerating epithelial cells increases the osmotic pressure which is instrumental in inducing a cystic structure, since this causes ingress of fluid into the cyst (1). Cysts increase in size by osmotic tension (4). A modified classification is as follows:

### NON-ODONTOGENIC CYSTS

| | |
|---|---|
| FISSURAL | Medial Palatine |
| | Median alveolar |
| | Globulomaxillary |
| | Median mandibular |
| VESTIGAL | Nasopalatine |
| | Nasopalatine duct |
| | Cyst of the papillapalatine |
| TRAUMATIC | Hemorrhagic |
| | Aneurysmal |

### ODONTOGENIC CYSTS

| | |
|---|---|
| FOLLICULAR | Primordial |
| | Dentigerous |
| LAMINAL | Odontogenic keratocyst |
| RADICULAR | Apical |
| | Periodontal |
| | Residual |

## Non Odontogenic Cysts

*Fissural Cysts*

These result from ectoderm residues in the formation of the facial skeleton. Particularly, epithelial rests at the lines of fusion tend to form cysts. The maxilla, at points of embryonic fusions, is a common site for cyst development from epithelial debris. The overall commonest site by far is the palatal midline. Cysts which occur anteriorly, behind the lingula aspect of the upper incisor teeth are termed medial alveolar cysts; if more posteriorly, medial palatal cysts (Fig. 1 a, b). Medial palatal cysts are usually located behind the incisive papilla, have an epithelial lined sac, are asymptomatic and on radiographs appear as a spherical radiolucent area (5) (Fig. 2). The alveolar medial cyst occurs between the roots of the central incisors.

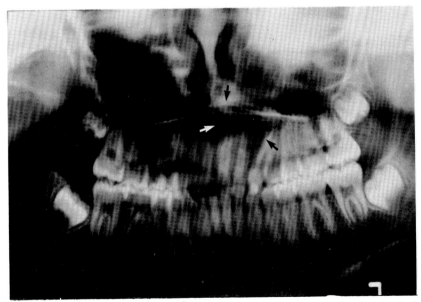

Figure 1a. Location behind incisive papilla midline position and spherical radiolucent shape, suggest that it is a medial palatal cyst.

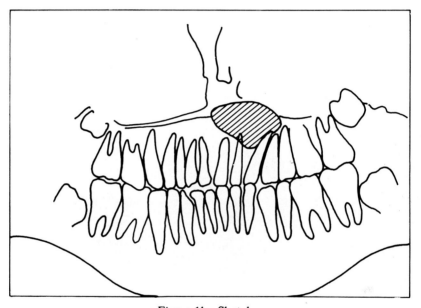

Figure 1b. Sketch.

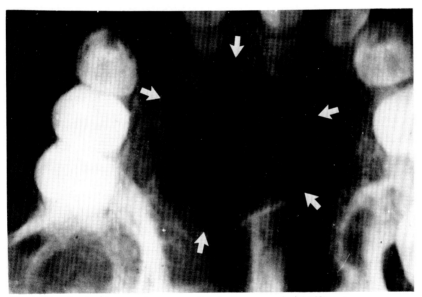

Figure 2. Occlusal view shows ovoid radiolucent cyst in the midline extending somewhat to the right.

The lateral bone inclusion cysts (Globulomaxillary) form at the site of fusion of the globular and maxillary processes of the maxillae. These globulomaxillary cysts appear between the roots of the upper lateral maxillary incisors and canine teeth and may extend to the maxillary antrum. They are well circumscribed and have an inverted pear shape (6). As the cyst grows, it may destroy part of the premaxilla. These cysts are not in direct association with tooth roots although during growth may encroach to distort the position of the cuspid and lateral incisor teeth (Fig. 3 a, b, c, d). Other lesions such as odontogenic keratocyst, radicular cyst and adenoid cystic carcinoma have been reported as simulating a globulomaxillary cyst (6).

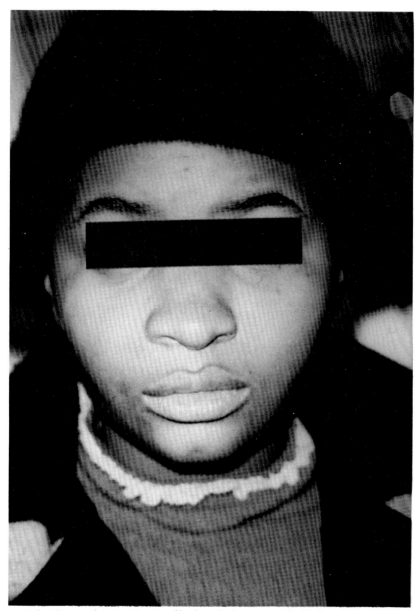

Figure 3a. Adolescent girl with swelling of the midline involving the lip.

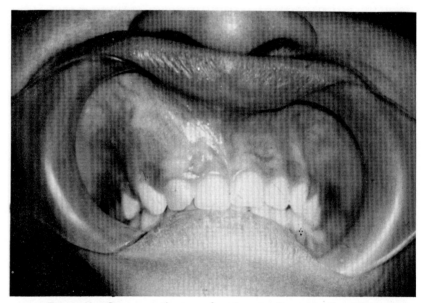

Figure 3b.  Open mouth view of cyst protruding onto the right.

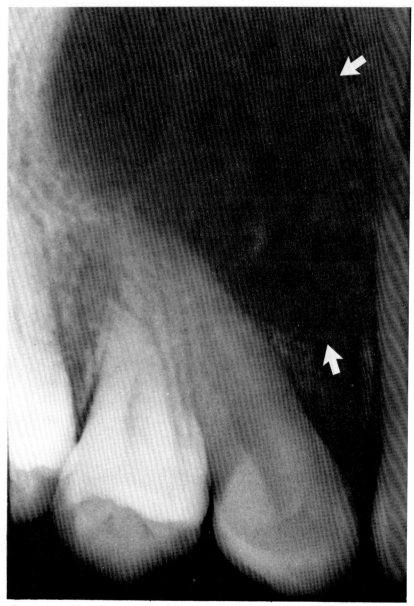

Figure 3c. Closeup radiograph shows a pear shaped globulomaxillary cyst.

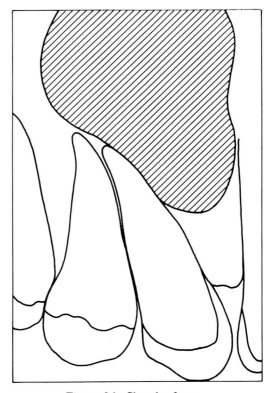

Figure 3d. Sketch of cyst.

*Vestigial Cysts*

Nasopalatine cysts are classified as incisive canal cysts and cysts of the papilla palatine. Incisive canal cysts are located high in the maxillary process. They originate from remnants of the nasopalatine ducts (7). An anterior view is needed to separate this lesion from the medial alveolar cyst (Fig. 4 a, b). The nasopalatine cyst is always at the midline and may be round or ovoid (Fig. 5 a, b). Expansion of the lesion follows the lines of least resistance; when the cyst expands to either side of the nasal spine it may assume a heart shape (Fig. 5 a, b), (Fig. 6 a, b) (7). The nasopalatine cyst may occur at any age but is more common after the age of 40.

The radiographic differentiation of this cyst from normal anatomic structures may sometimes be difficult. An incisive fossa up to 0.6 cms. in width is considered normal (8). The cysts are located between, or above the roots of the central incisors sometime appearing as periapical pathology. Also, the margins of a cyst are more well defined, more spherical and higher than the fossa (9). These cysts may present with pain, particularly if they become infected (10).

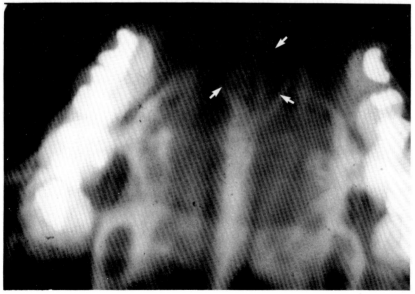

Figure 4a. An ovoid cyst at midline originating from the nasopalatine duct *(arrows)*.

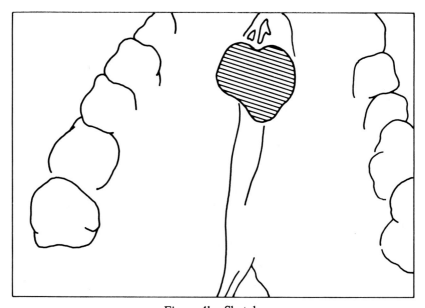

Figure 4b. Sketch.

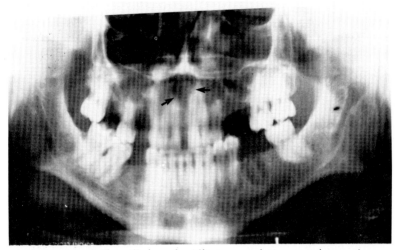

Figure 5a. A "heart" shaped midline nasopalatine cyst *(arrows)*.

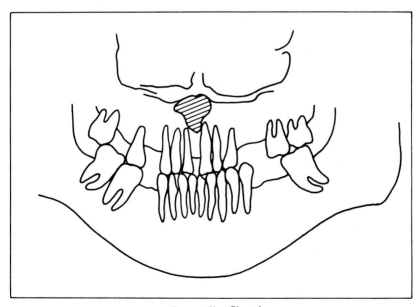

Figure 5b. Sketch.

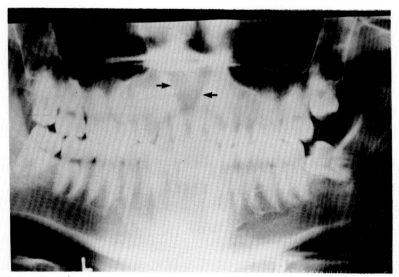

Figure 6a. On a panorex the triangular shape of a nasopalatine cyst *(arrows)* is accentuated.

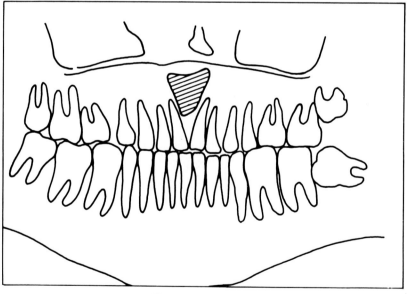

Figure 6b. Sketch.

### Odontogenic Cysts

The lining of most of these cysts is stratified squamous epithelium. In the maxillary antrum cysts may be lined by respiratory epithelium. The cyst wall is usually formed by fibrous tissue. Also, in the event that hemorrhage has occurred, macrophages or giant cell reaction may be observed.

Follicular cysts surround the crowns of impacted teeth (11) and they have their origin from defective development of the tooth (12). There are many classifications; most include primordial cyst and dentigerous cyst, some odontogenic keratocyst. These all derive from dental organ epithelium. The primordial cyst forms in the tooth bud before mature ameloblasts or hard tissue appear. These commonly occur in the mandibular third molar, and may surround the crowns of impacted teeth; if the tooth bud is involved and becomes cystic the molar will be missing. The radiographic appearance is not specific; usually there is a missing permanent tooth (10). These cysts also occur at the level of maxillary and mandibular canines. On radiographs, they are well defined radiolucencies and, again, may be seen where there are absent teeth. They are outlined by thin radiopaque borders and may be multiloculated. The primordial cyst occurs most commonly before 30 years of age. They frequently prove to be keratocysts on histologic examinations. The primordial cyst may also be confused with residual cyst (Fig. 7 a, b). This occurs most commonly in the mandible in edentulous areas. It is a follicular cyst remaining after a tooth extraction (Fig. 8 a).

In cases of multiple basal cell nevus syndrome where odontogenic keratocysts is a component, Gorlin has reported a prediliction towards transformation of this cyst into ameloblastoma (13).

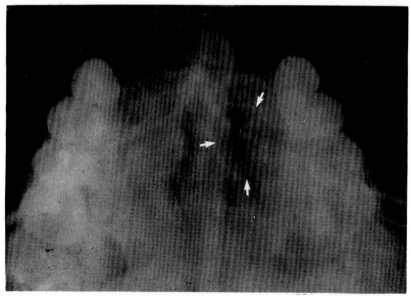

Figure 7a. A residual cyst off midline *(arrows)*. Radiographic appearance is not specific. Missing teeth suggest origin.

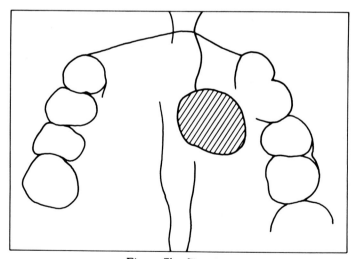

Figure 7b. Sketch.

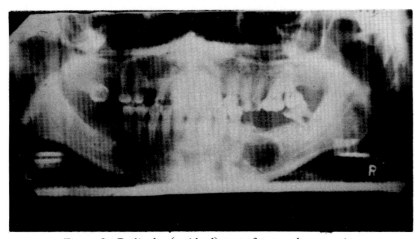

Figure 8.  Radicular (residual) cyst after tooth extraction.

Dentigerous cysts occur in the later stages of tooth development and are associated with the crown of an unerupted tooth. They are usually found between the ages of 13-40 years (14). Most frequently they occur as a complication of impacted molars where normal eruption has been impeded;(Fig. 9 a, b) and (Fig. 10 a, b), the mandibular third molar is the commonest site (15). They can also occur at the sites of the maxillary canines (Fig. 11 a, b) or mandibular premolars. Dentigerous cysts often expand rapidly and can cause maxillary sinus involvement if they occur in the maxillary canine area (Fig. 12 a, b).

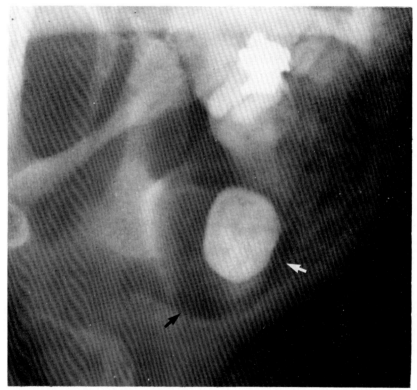

Figure 9a. Cystic area in the left mandible with retained tooth *(arrows)*. This proved to be a dentigerous cyst.

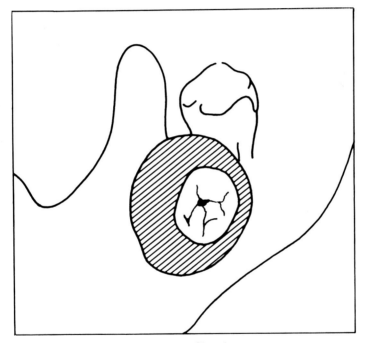

Figure 9b. Sketch.

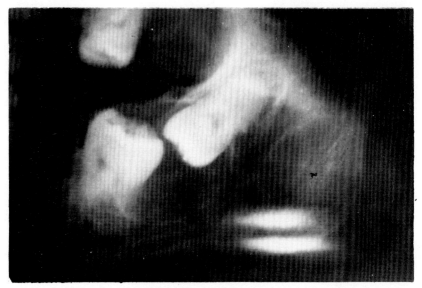

Figure 10a. Dentigerous cyst of the angle of the mandible.

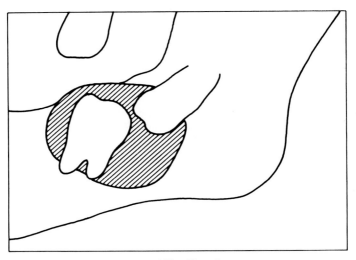

Figure 10b. Sketch.

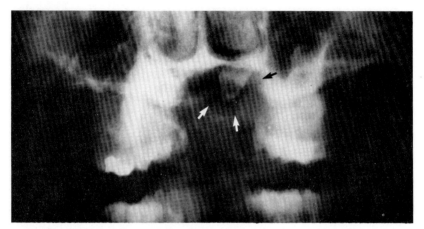

Figure 11a. A dentigerous cyst at the maxillary cuspid *(arrows)*.

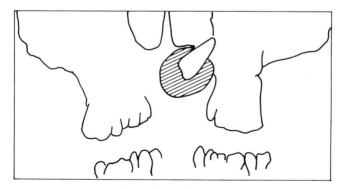

Figure 11b. Sketch.

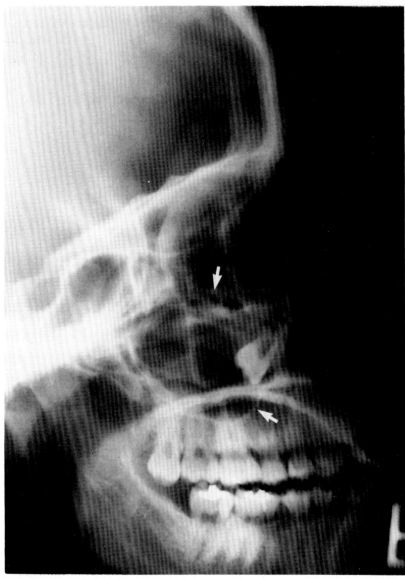

Figure 12a. Dentigerous cyst with impacted molar in its wall *(arrows)*. The maxillary sinus is eroded, and the entire crown of the tooth is involved.

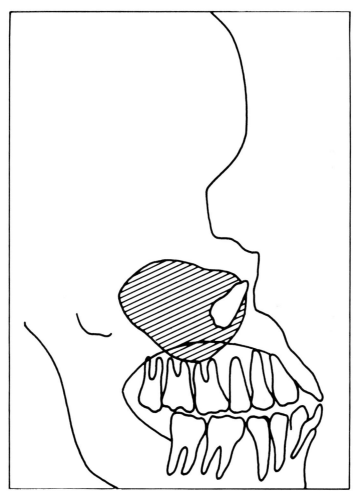

Figure 12b. Sketch.

On radiographs, the entire tooth crown may be involved (central type) (Fig. 13 a, b, c), or only part of the crown (lateral type). Sometimes the presence of a tooth crown pointing towards the center of the cyst helps to differentiate it from primordial cysts. However, when the cyst becomes very large, the molar may be displaced along the cyst wall so that differentiating it from a primordial cyst becomes more difficult. The width of the pericoronal space exceeding 1 mm may be the earliest clue to a developing dentigerous cyst (14). Careful histological examination of excised cyst walls should be carried out since neoplastic potentials have been associated with dentigerous cysts (16-19). In Gardner's review of the literature he found 63 cases of squamous cell carcinoma which had its origin in an odontogenic cyst (20). He found 25 cases that were acceptable instances, and among these the median age was 57. A rapid increase in jaw size was an important clinical finding. Failure of the extraction site to heal, displacement of teeth and appearance of a flat or papilliferous mass attached to the base at the time of enucleation were also presenting features. On radiographs, the radiolucencies in the jaw had ill defined, jagged indented borders and roots of teeth adjacent to the radiolucent area showed resorption. Bony expansion with cortical thinning was common (20).

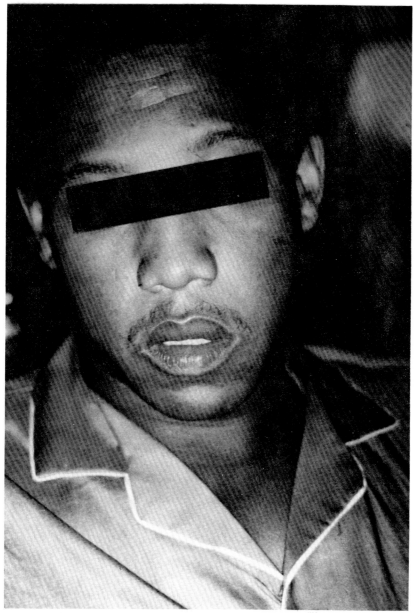

Figure 13a. Swelling of the cheek in a young black male.

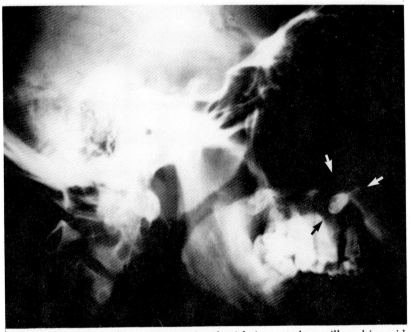

Figure 13b. Dentigerous cyst associated with impacted maxillary bicuspid; on lateral view tooth appears central in the cyst *(arrows)*.

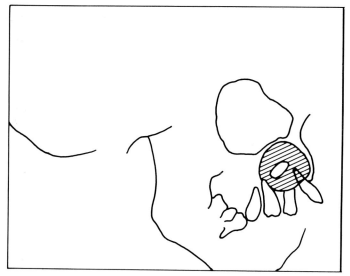

Figure 13c. Sketch.

The odontogenic keratocyst is classified distinct from other cysts because of its histological appearance. These also have previously been called primordial cysts since both have a thin wall of keratinizing epithelium on histology (Fig. 14 a, b). In Rud's series, 2/3 of the patients with odontogenic keratocysts were less than 40 years of age (11). The peak incidence occurs in the second decade (10).

Most lesions occur at the level of the mandibular third molar or maxillary canine. The radiographic appearance is similar to that of nonkeratinized cysts, and cannot be distinguished from other cysts by means of x-ray examinations. If there is a haziness (due to the keratin filling the cyst) within a hyperostic border, the diagnosis of keratocyst may be suspected. They may also be large and multilocular and resemble an ameloblastoma.

Radicular cysts and apical periodontal cysts (Radicular cysts, periapical cyst). These are common lesions and are caused by inflammation of the dental pulp and periodontal membrane. Remnants of Hertwig's sheath are trapped in resulting granulomas formation and the epithelial rests proliferate to line the cyst. These appear as small areas of radiolucency about the roots of a tooth. In the maxilla, it is usually anterior in location; in the mandible posterior (22-28).

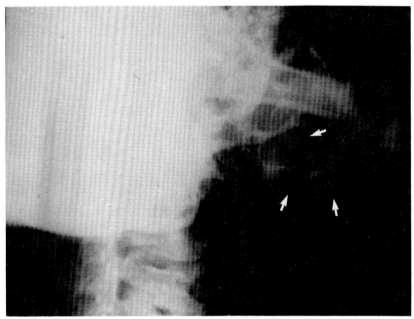

Figure 14a. Numerous keratocysts of the mandibular ramus area *(arrows)*.

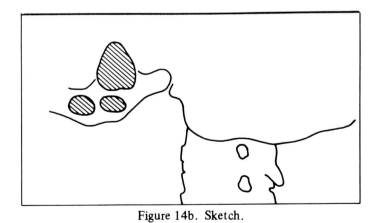

Figure 14b. Sketch.

When the cyst occurs at the tooth apex, it is called periapical. If the cyst is not identified at the time of tooth extraction and appears afterwards, it is called a residual cyst (Figs. 7, 8). However, those oriented along the lateral surface of the tooth are classified lateral periodontal cysts. On x-ray, a sharply outlined radiolucent cyst rimmed by a margin of dense cortical bone is seen (Fig. 15). Adjacent structures may be displaced.

It is not always possible to distinguish a periapical granuloma from a radicular cyst on basis of radiographic examination alone (Fig. 16 a, b, c, d). To separate the two, cysts are generally held to be well circumscribed and at least 10 mms in diameter, and outlined by a thin even white layer of cortical bone (24). Periapical granulomas seldom exceed 1 cm in diameter and usually do not have a white line surrounding the area of radiolucency.

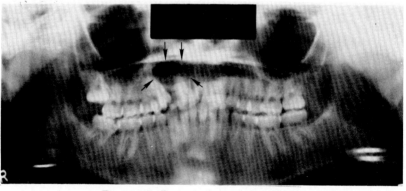

Figure 15. Periapical cyst in maxilla.

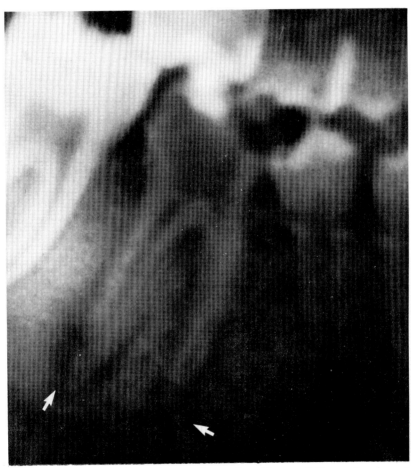

Figure 16a. Periapical granulomas. Lucencies at base of the molar do not exceed 1 cm. in diameter and do not have a white line surrounding the area of lucency *(arrows)*. The crown is carious.

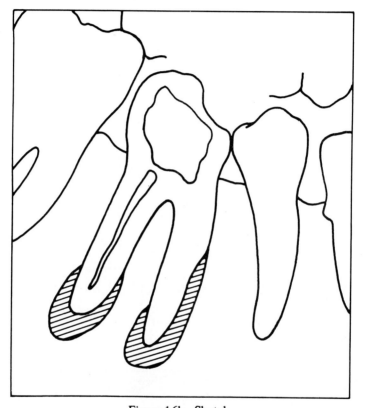

Figure 16b. Sketch.

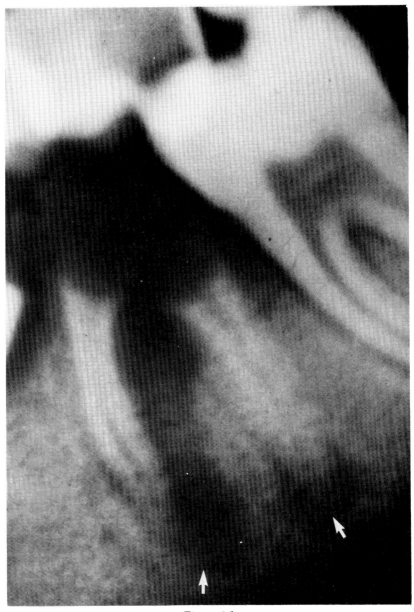

Figure 16c.

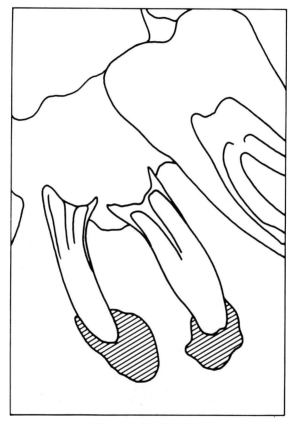

Figure 16d. Sketch.

## References

1. Spouge, J.D.: Oral Pathology. C.V. Mosby Co. St. Louis, 1973, pp. 302-320.
2. Main, D.M.G.: Epithelial jaw cysts. A clinicopathological reappraisal. Br. J. Oral Surg., 8:114-125, 1970.
3. Stafne, E.C.: Oral Roentgenographic Diagnosis, 3rd ed. W.B. Saunders Co. Philadelphia, p. 147.
4. Toller, P.A.: Newer concepts of odontogenic cysts. Int. J. Oral Surg., 1:3-16, 1972.
5. Thornton, W.C., Allen, J.W., and Byrd, D.L.: Median palatal cyst: Report of case. J. Oral Surg., 30:661-663, 1973.
6. Zegarelli, D.J., and Zegarelli, E.V.: Radiolucent lesions in the globulo-maxillary region. J. Oral Surg., 31:767-771, 1973.
7. Campbell, J.J., Baden, E., and Williams, A.C.: Nasopalatine cyst of unusual size: Report of case. J. Oral Surg., 31:776-779, 1973.
8. Abrams, A.M., Howell, F.V., and Bullock, W.K.: Nasopalatine cyst. Oral Surg., 16:306-332, 1963.
9. Stafne, E.C., Austine, L.T., and Gardner, B.S.: Median anterior maxillary cyst. J. Am. Dent. Assoc., 23:801-809, 1936.
10. Wood, N.K., and Goaz, P.W.: Differential Diagnosis of Oral Lesions. C.V. Mosby Co. 1975, pp. 319-330.
11. Rud, J., and Pindborg, J.J.: Odontogenic keratocysts: A follow-up study of 21 cases. J. Oral Surg., 27:323-330, 1969.
12. Jaffe, H.L.: Tumors and Tumorous Conditions of the Bones and Joints. Lea and Febiger, Philadelphia, 1958, pp. 425-435.
13. Gorlin, R.J., Vickers, R.A., Relln, E., and Williamson, J.J.: The multiple basal cell nevi syndrome. Cancer, 18:890104, 1965.
14. Mourshed, F.: A roentgenographic study of dentigerous cysts. Oral Surg., 18:47-53, 1964.
15. Fickling, B.W.: Cysts of the jaw. A long term survey of types and treatment. Proc. Roy. Soc. Med., 58:847-854, 1965.
16. Stanley, H.R., and Biehl, D.L.: Ameloblastoma potential of follicular cysts. Oral Surg., 20:260-269, 1965.
17. Gorlin, R.J.: Potentialities of oral epithelium manifest by mandibular dentigerous cysts. Oral Surg., 10:271-284, 1957.
18. Eversole, L.R., Sabes, W.R., and Rovin, S.: Aggressive growth and neoplastic potential of odontogenic cysts. Cancer, 35:270-282, 1975.
19. Giansanti, J.S., Someren, A., and Waldron, C.A.: Odontogenic adenomatoid tumor (adenoameloblastoma). Oral Surg., 30:69-86, 1970.
20. Gardner, A.F.: The odontogenic cyst as a potential carcinoma: A clinicopathologic appraisal. J. Am. Dent. Assoc., 78:746-755, 1969.

21. Enriquez, R.E., Ciola, B., and Bahn, S.L.: Verrucous carcinoma arising in an odontogenic cyst: Report of case. Oral Surg., 49:151-156, 1980.
22. Abrams, A.M., and Howell, F.V.: The calcifying odontogenic cyst. Oral Surg., 25:594-606, 1968.
23. Priebe, W.A., Lazansky, J.P., and Wuehrmann, A.H.: The value of the roentgenographic film in the differential diagnosis of periapical lesions. Oral Surg., 7:979-983, 1954.
24. Linenberg, W.B., Waldron, C.A., and Delaune, G.F.: A clinical roentgenographic and histopathologic evaluation of periapical lesions. Oral Surg., 17:467-472, 1964.
25. Bhasker, S.N.: Periapical lesions-types, incidence, and clinical features. Oral Surg., 21:657-671, 1966.
26. Oehler, F.A.C.: Periapical lesions and residual dental cysts. Br. J. Oral Surg., 8:103-113, 1970.
27. Lalonde, E.R., and Luebke, R.G.: The frequency and distribution of periapical cysts and granulomas. Oral Surg., 25:861-868, 1968.
28. Mortensen, H., Winther, J.E., and Birn, H.: Periapical granulomas and cysts. Scand. J., Dent. Res., 78:241-250, 1970.

## TRAUMATIC BONE CYST

Traumatic bone cyst is not actually a cyst since it does not have an epithelial lining. The pathogenesis is not clear but may represent an area of bony injury, sufficient to rupture blood vessels with ensuing hemorrhage. The intraosseous blood clot liquifies or resorbs so that the cavity will either be filled with straw colored fluid or remnant of blood clots. The specimen will consequently contain no epithelial lining, and, loose connective tissue containing granulation tissue and giant cells may line the bone adjacent to the cavity (1).

Local forces of injury may produce a subperiosteal hematoma, followed by destruction of the blood supply and accentuated osteoclastic activity. A deficit will remain when this activity regresses (2). Hemorrhage into a cyst has been shown to cause a rise in cyst pressure which, in a confined bony space, may contribute to pressure atrophy of the cyst wall, intermittent small hemorrhage and slow expansion (3).

This cyst occurs in young patients, most in adolescents and young adults (1). It is somewhat more common in men than women, by 3:1; it almost always occurs in the mandible (1, 4, 6), where the premolar-molar area is most frequent site. The lesion usually is not associated with pain. Few cases presenting with pain or trismus are described (7). It has also been referred to as a simple cyst, hemorrhagic bone cyst or latent extravasation cyst (8). Multiple adjacent cysts, presumably before expanding into one cavity have been described (9). Bilateral traumatic cysts although uncommon have been reported. Routine radiographic screening suggest that it is probably more common than previously reported (8).

On radiographs, it appears as a radiolucent well defined area above the inferior dental canal. The lamina dura of adjacent teeth usually remains intact although the cyst may impinge on the roots (Fig. 17 a, b). The outline may be irregular or follow the outline of the jaw bone (10). The roots of adjacent teeth may extend into the cyst (2), which produces a scalloped defect between and around the roots of the teeth (4, 5).

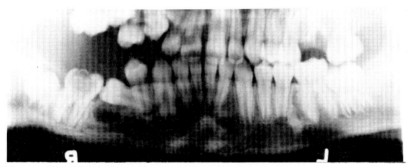

Figure 17a. Bi-lobed cystic area beneath incisors, bicuspids and molar extending toward the midline. This appeared after trauma.

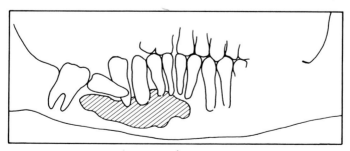

Figure 17b. Sketch.

## References

*Traumatic Bone Cyst*

1. Heubner, G.R., and Turlington, E.G.: So called traumatic (hemorrhagic) bone cysts of the jaws. Oral Surg., 31:354-365, 1971.
2. Bernier, J.L.: Tumors of the odontogenic apparatus and jaws. AFIP Atlas of Tumor Pathology. Section IV, Fascicle 10A. Washington, D.C., 1960.
3. Toller, P.A.: Radioactive isotope and other investigations in a case of haemorrhagic cyst of the mandible: Br. J. Oral Surg., 86-93, 1964.
4. Howe, G.: "Haemorrhagic cysts" of the mandible I., II Br. J. Oral Surg., 11:55-76, 1965; 11:77-91, 1965.
5. Stewart, S., Sherman, P., and Stoopack, J.C.: Large bilateral traumatic bone cysts of the mandible: Report of case. Oral Surg., 31:865-868, 1973.
6. Fickling, B.W.: Cysts of the jaw: A long-term survey of types and treatment. Proc. Roy. Soc. Med., 58:847-854, 1965.
7. Daramola, J.O., Samuel, I., Ajaqbe, H.A., and Kahn, S.: Traumatic cyst of the mandible. J. Oral Surg., 36:282-284, 1978.
8. Morris, C.R., Steed, D.L., and Jacoby, J.J.: Traumatic bone cysts. J. Oral Surg., 28:188-195, 1970.
9. Schofeld, I.D.F.: An unusual traumatic bone cyst. Oral Surg., 38:198-203, 1974.
10. Ivy, R., and Curtis, L.: Hemorrhagic or traumatic cysts of mandible. Surg. Gynecol., Obstet., 65:640-643, 1937.

## ANEURYSMAL BONE CYST

Aneurysmal bone cyst was first described by Jaffe and Lichtenstein in 1942 (1). These cysts are benign, causing local expansion and occur predominantly in the spine and long bones and only rarely in the jaws (2). The cysts occur mostly in adolescents and young adults with no sex predominance. When found in the jaw bones, the lesion is seen more often in the mandible than the maxilla (3-5).

Untreated, these cysts grow in size at varying rates. Clinically, the jaw will have a swelling at the site of the lesion, which will be fusiform or round and of firm consistency. Rapid growth of the lesion has been demonstrated in aneurysmal bone cysts elsewhere in the body (6). On occasion, it may be associated with a tooth extraction or other injury in young patients (9). Trauma, although often part of the clinical history, has (7) not proven to be directly related (8).

The etiology is not known but is thought to be related to an arteriovenous aneurysm or venous thrombosis with subsequent increase in venous pressure and development of an engorged vascular bed. Resorption of bone by giant cells ensues which is replaced by connective tissue and new bone (1). Another pathogenesis described relates initial medullary hemorrhage whereby the aneurysmal bone cyst is thought to represent an attempt by connective tissue to repair the hematoma in the marrow. If there is a maintained connection with damaged blood vessels, then an aneurysmal bone cyst results (7, 8). Only a few documented cases of preceding trauma are described (10). Continuous pulsation from the blood vessels will expand the mandible only when the main vessels connect to the hematoma. If minor vessels are connected to the hematoma, then repair will lead to capillary budding, formation of groups of giant cells and a giant cell granuloma will be produced (7, 11). Arteriovenous fistulas have been demonstrated by angiography, histological examination and by documenting, within the cyst cavities elevated vascular pressures (12). An expansile fistula eroding, and resorbing adjacent bone can produce a pathological picture similar to aneurysmal bone cyst (12).

On histological examination, bone is replaced by spongy fibro-osseous tissue which contain blood filled cavernous vessels (13). Variable numbers of channels do not have the elastic tissue or muscle found in blood vessels but often consist of collagenous material, immature bone trabeculae and giant cells (14, 15) (Fig. 18 d).

On radiographs, the jaw is expanded into a thinned out shell of bone (Fig. 18 a, b, c, d). This shell may be defective in places and is often convoluted (16). Within this are faintly outlined radiolucencies which may be hazy and mottled or with a fine trabecular pattern growing coarser towards the edges of the lesion, producing a honeycombed or soap bubble appearance (17, 18), not unlike hemangioma or myxoma (Fig. 19 a, b, c, d).

Radiographs may not always prove to be diagnostic and ameloblastoma, follicular cyst, traumatic cyst or other cyst must be considered (5, 7, 13).

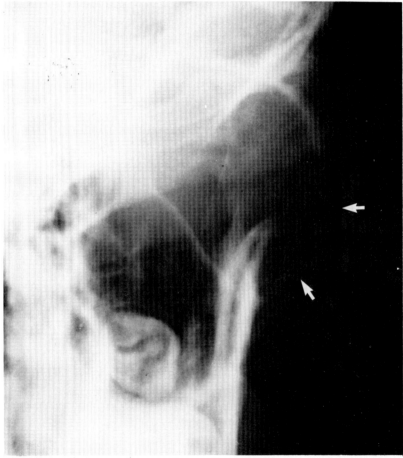

Figure 18a. Apparent absence of ascending ramus and condyle of mandible. There is an apparent cystic expansion *(arrows).*

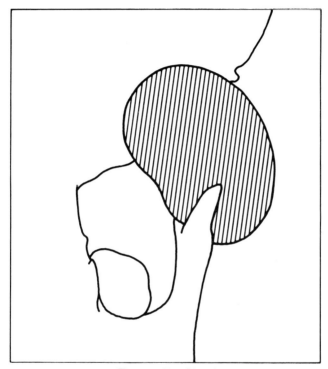

Figure 18b. Sketch.

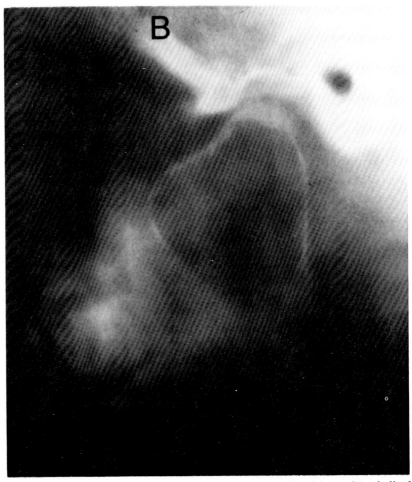

Figure 18c. Laminograph shows expanded ramus outlined by a thin shell of bone. This proved to be an aneurysmal bone cyst.

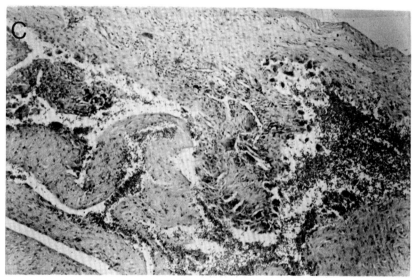

Figure 18d. Histology demonstrates blood filled spaces outlined by fibrous tissue septa with many multinucleated giant cells along their lining.

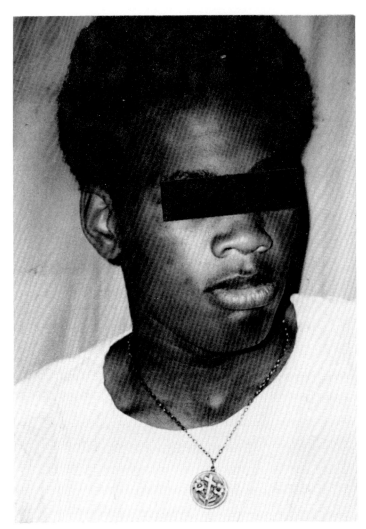

Figure 19a. A 15-year-old black male presented with swelling on the chin.

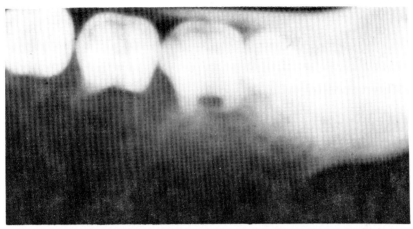

Figure 19b. On anterioposterior view there are faintly outlined radiolucencies within the cyst producing a honeycombed appearance and enlargement of the lateral cortex.

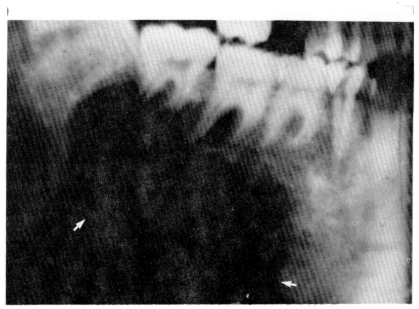

Figure 19c. There is expansion by the aneurysmal bone cyst and there is scalloping around roots of the molar teeth *(arrows)*.

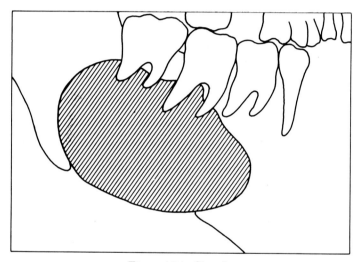

Figure 19d. Sketch.

## References

1. Jaffe, H.L., and Lichtenstein, L.: Solitary unicameral bone cyst, with emphasis on the roentgen picture, the pathologic appearance and the pathogenesis. Arch. Surg., 44:1004-1025, 1942.
2. Killey, H.C., and Kay, L.W.: Benign Cystic Lesions of the Jaws. Their Diagnosis and Treatment. E. and S. Livingstone. London, 1966, pp. 104-106.
3. Byrd, D.L., Allen, J.W., Kindrick, R.D., and DeWitt, J.D.: Aneurysmal bone cyst of the maxilla. J. Oral Surg., 27:296-300, 1969.
4. Daugherty, J.W., and Eversole, L.R.: Aneurysmal bone cyst of the mandible: Report of case. J. Oral Surg., 29:737-741, 1971.
5. Gruskin, S.E., and Dahlin, D.C.: Aneurysmal bone cysts of the jaws: J. Oral Surg., 26:523-528, 1968.
6. Clough, J.R., and Price, C.H.G.: Aneurysmal bone cysts. Review of 12 cases. JBJS, 50B:116-127, 1968.
7. Bhaskar, S.N., Bernier, J.L., and Godby, F.: Aneurysmal bone cyst and other giant cell lesions of the jaws: Report of 104 cases. J. Oral Surg., 17:30-41, 1959.
8. Romaniuk, K., and Becker, R.: Two cases of aneurysmal bone cysts of the jaws. Int. J. Oral Surg., 1:48-52, 1972.
9. Bernier, J.L.: Tumors of the odontogenic apparatus and jaws. AFIP Atlas of Tumor Pathology, section IV, Fascicle, 10A Washington, D.C., 1960.
10. Reyneke, J.P.: Aneurysmal bone cyst of the maxilla. Oral Surg., 45:441-447, 1978.
11. Hillerup, S., and Hjorting-Hansen, E.: Aneurysmal bone cyst-simple bone cyst, two aspects of the same pathologic entity? Int. J. Oral Surg., 7:16-22, 1978.
12. Biesecker, J.L., Marcove, R.C., Huvos, A.G., and Mike, V.: Aneurysmal bone cysts. A clinico-pathological study of 66 cases. Cancer, 26:615-628, 1970.
13. Oliver, L.P.: Aneurysmal bone cyst. Oral Surg., 35:67-76, 1973.
14. Tillman, B.P., Dahlin, D.C., Lipscomb, P.R., and Stewart, J.R.: Aneurysmal bone cyst: An analysis of ninety-five cases. Mayo Clin. Proc., 43:478-495, 1968.
15. Lichtenstein, L.: Aneurysmal bone cyst. Observations of fifty cases. JBJS, 39:873-882, 1968.
16. Sharp, G.W., Bullock, W.K., and Hazlet, J.W.: Oral Cancer and Tumors of the Jaws. McGraw Hill. New York, 1956. pp. 505-509.
17. Dahlin, D.C., Besse, B.E., Pugh, D.G., and Ghormley, R.K.: Aneurysmal bone cysts. Radiology, 64:56-65, 1955.

# 3

## ODONTOGENIC TUMORS

### AMELOBLASTOMA

The origin of its name reflects the fact that the histological appearance of the tumor cell resembles those of developing enamel organ. However, there is no evidence that the tumor originates from the ameloblast although the nomenclature has persevered. The ameloblastoma is composed of epithelium and develops from epithelial cells in one of multiple locations (1). The tumor probably arises from the basal cell of the oral epithelium (2).

The tumor is rare, occuring in only 1% of all jaw bone tumors and cysts (3). Analysis of over 100 cases by Small and Waldron showed that the most common age group was 20-40 years. This age distribution was also recorded by Robinson (4), by Masson (5) and by Hertz (6). Ameloblastoma is most uncommon in children, (3, 7) and may be of a different cell type than adults (7).

There is controversy as to whether the ameloblastoma can arise from a dentigerous cyst despite well documented cases. Stanley and Diehl studied 108 cases of ameloblastoma associated with a cyst and noted that there was a decrease in incidence of the two in association after 30 years of age (8). Castner (9) described an 11-year-old girl who had a pathologically confirmed ameloblastoma arising in a follicular cyst (9).

The tumor arises in the mandible in 80% of the cases (3, 5, 10), most in the molar area or near the angle of the mandible (11). About 10% are associated with an unerupted tooth in the cyst lumen (5). Ameloblastomas which appear in the maxilla are more common in the cuspid area and may extend into the maxillary sinus, nose or orbit. In a recent study, the majority of tumors involving the maxilla were located in the posterior maxilla and 50% of the patients had maxillary antrum involvement (12). Radiographic appearance in this location is not characteristic (11). Because of its invasive nature and its tendency to recur (Fig. 20), ameloblastoma is considered to have malignant potential (5) (Fig. 21 a, b, c, d).

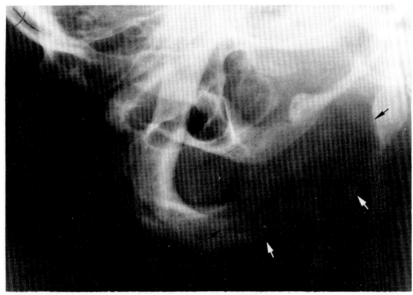

Figure 20a. Conedown from frontal view of the mandible in an edentulous patient. The wavy contour of the inner aspect of the mandible suggests an ameloblastoma *(arrows)*. This tumor recurred twice.

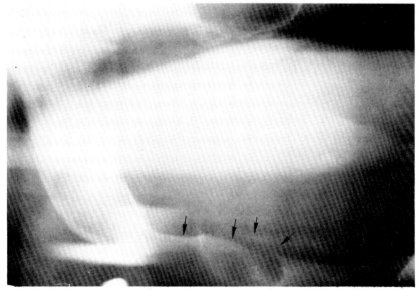

Figure 20b. Oblique view of the mandible shows extent of the tumor *(arrows)*.

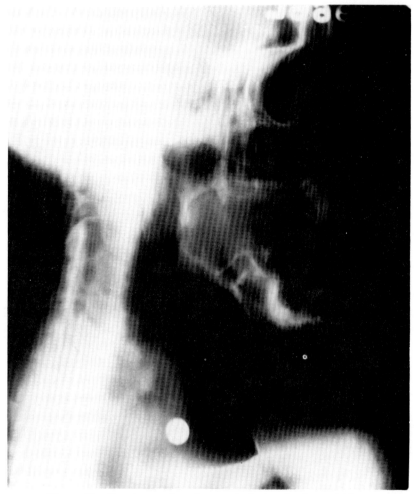

Figure 21a. Laminography of extensively involved mandible.

Figure 21a-d. Three examples of ameloblastoma. All have scalloped wavy borders.

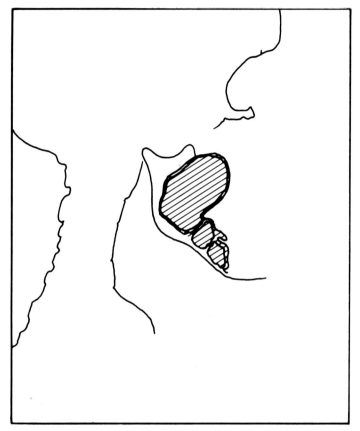

Figure 21b. Sketch.

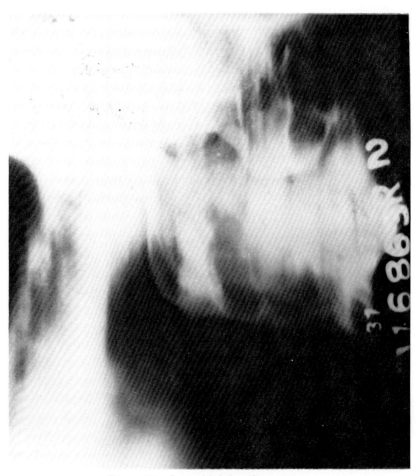

Figure 21c. Large Multilocular tumor.

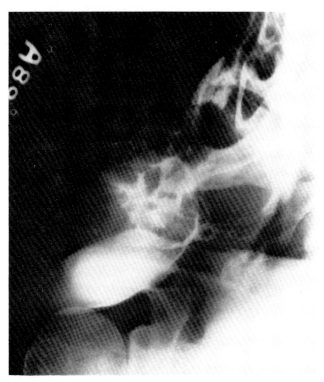

Figure 21d. Giant ameloblastoma extending in an exophytic manner (courtesy Dr. E. Espinoza, Westside V.A. Hospital, Chicago).

On radiographs, the classic appearance is that of multilocular radio-lucencies associated with local expansion. In some cases, when there is a tooth present, the tumor will appear as a mononuclear bone defect, and differen-tiation from a dentigerous cyst may be difficult (Fig. 22 a, b). Differential diagnosis includes fibrous dysplasia, hemorrhagic bone cysts, odontogenic tumors, mxyoma, salivary gland tumors and histiocystosis X.

The tumor spreads into the cancellous space without bony resorption. This bone may appear normal on radiographs and at surgery. However, the ameloblastoma does not invade the Haversian canals or compact bone. In the compact bone at the inferior border of the mandible, radiographs show the true tumor extension (13). There have been a few well documented cases of malignant ameloblastoma (14). Metastases to the lungs (15, 16, 17), local lymph nodes or vertebral body metastasis (18, 19) occur when the tumor is of long duration with local spread and when there have been multiple operations or radiation therapy.

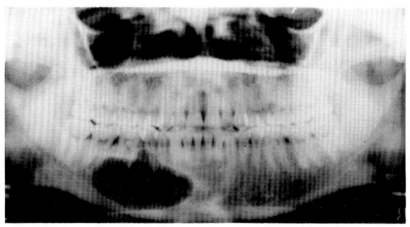

Figure 22a. An ameloblastoma appearing as an unilocular cavity having the appearance of an odontogenic cyst. Roots of cuspid and molar teeth are splayed.

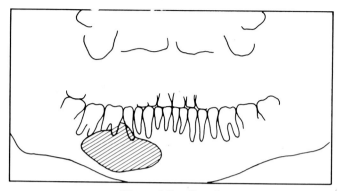

Figure 22b. Sketch.

## References

*Ameloblastoma*

1. Gorlin, R.J., Chaudhry, A.P., and Pindborg, J.J.: Odontogenic tumors classification, histopathology and clinical behavior in man and domesticated animals. Cancer, 14:73-101, 1961.
2. Smith, J.F.: The controversial ameloblastoma. Oral Surg., 26:45-75, 1968.
3. Small, I.A., and Waldron, C.A.: Ameloblastomas of the jaws. Oral Surg., 8:281-297, 1955.
4. Robinson, H.B.G.: Ameloblastoma: A survey of 379 cases from the literature. Arch Path., 23:831-843, 1937.
5. Masson, J.K., McDonald, J.R., and Figi, F.A.: Adamantinoma of the jaws: A clinicopathologic study of 101 histologically proved cases. Plast. Reconstr. Surg., 23:510-525, 1959.
6. Hertz, J.: Adamantinoma. Histo-pathologic and Prognostic studies. Acta Chir Scand., 102:405-432, 1952.
7. Young, D.R., and Robinson, M.: Ameloblastomas in children. Oral Surg., 15:1155-1162, 1962.
8. Stanley, H.R., and Diehl, D.L.: Ameloblastoma potential of follicular cysts. Oral Surg., 20:260-268, 1965.
9. Castner, D.V., McCully, A.C., and Hiatt, W.R.: Intracystic ameloblastoma in the young patient. Oral Surg., 23:127-134, 1967.
10. Adekeye, E.O.: Ameloblastoma of the jaws: A survey of 109 Nigerian patients. J. Oral Surg., 38:36-41, 1980.
11. Spouge, J.D.: Oral Pathology. C.V. Mosby Co. St. Louis, 1973, pp. 321-331.
12. Tsaknis, P.J., and Nelson, J.F.: The maxillary ameloblastoma: An analysis of 24 cases. J. Oral Surg., 38:336-338, 1980.

13. Kramer, I.R.H.: Ameloblastoma: A clinicopathological appraisal. Br. J. Oral Surg., 1:13-28, 1963.

14. Carr, R.F., and Halperin, V.: Malignant ameloblastomas from 1953 to 1966. Oral Surg., 26:514-522, 1967.

15. Schweitzer, F.C., and Barnfield, W.F.: Ameloblastoma of the mandible with metastasis to the lungs. Report of a case. J. Oral Surg., 1:287-295, 1943.

16. Vorzimer, J., and Perla, D.: An instance of adamantinoma of the jaw with metastases to the right lung. Amer. J. Path., 8:445-454, 1943.

17. Tsukada, Y., Dela Pava, S., and Pickren, J.W.: Granular-cell ameloblastoma with metastasis to the lungs. Cancer, 18:916-925, 1965.

18. Hoke, H.F., and Harrelson, A.B.: Granular cell ameloblastoma with metastasis to the cervical vertebrae. Cancer, 20:991-999, 1967.

19. Sugimura, M., Yamauchi, T., Yashikawa, K., Takeda, N., Sakita, M., and Miyazaki, T.: Malignant ameloblastoma with metastasis to the lumbar vertebrae: Report of case. J. Oral Surg., 27:350-357, 1969.

## ADENO-AMELOBLASTOMA

This is a rare lesion with a more benign course than ameloblastoma. Various names are applied to this tumor: Ameloblastic adenomatoid tumor, Odontogenic mixed tumor, Adenomatoid odontogenic tumor. According to Tchertkoff, the tumor occurs in male/female patients with a ratio of 2:1 (1). Reviews by Gorlin (2) and by Bhaskar (3) state that the reverse is true and that females are predominant by 2:1. The most frequent site is the lateral incisor, cuspid area of the mandible or maxilla. Phillipsen demonstrated that 49 of 51 cases were in the anterior jaw region (4). Most patients seen in a series reported by Tchertkoff *et al.* were young, between 12-20 years of age (1). Association with an embedded tooth is seen in 75% of the cases (3) and suggests an odontogenic origin (Fig. 23 a, b, c, d, e).

On radiographs, these tumors generally appear as cystic radiolucent areas associated with unerupted teeth, and cannot always be distinguished from dentigerous cysts (Fig. 1). Among features differentiating them from dentigerous cysts are small irregular radiopacities which may be visible in the cyst like area (5, 6, 7), although these are not always present. The area of radiolucency surrounding the crown of the tooth is often to the side of the crown while dentigerous cysts surround the tooth symmetrically (5, 7). Also, when the lesion presents with a dentigerous cyst appearance, it can be differentiated since it extends apically beyond the cementoenamel junction (8, 7). However, diagnosis can only be confirmed on histological examination (1). Bhaskar believes that these tumors are follicular cysts with proliferation of its lining into the cyst cavity (3).

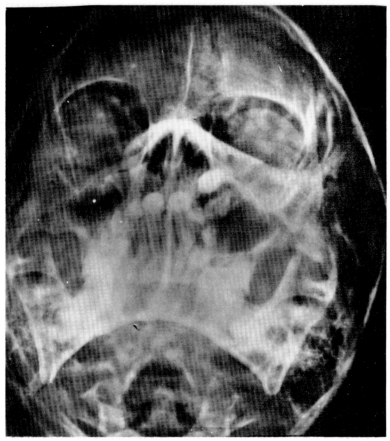

Figure 23a. Water's view: Many teeth are protruding from a radiolucent mass, extending into the left maxillary antrum. Histologically this was an ameloblastic adenomatoid tumor.

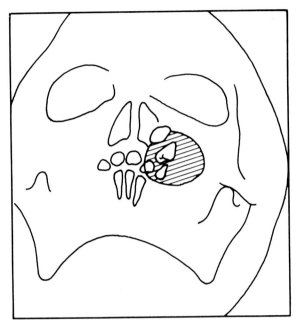

Figure 23b. Sketch.

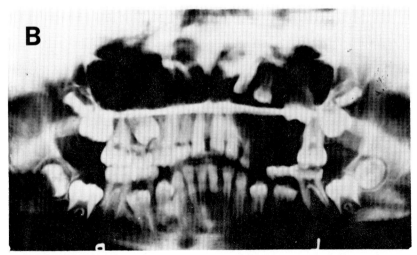

Figure 23c. Panorex more accurately delineates the size of the tumor.

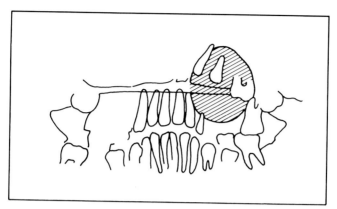

Figure 23d. Sketch.

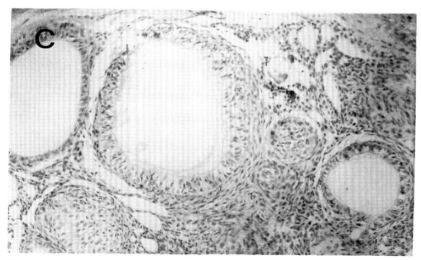

Figure 23e. Glandular spaces and solid walls of ameloblastic epithelial cells are shown (courtesy of Dr. Paul Szantos, Pathology Department, Cook County Hospital).

**References**

*Adenoameloblastoma*

1.  Tchertkoff, V., Daino, J.A., and Ehrenreich, T.: Ameloblastic adenomatoid tumor (adenoameloblastoma). Oral Surg., 27:72-82, 1969.
2.  Gorlin, R.J., Chaudhry, A.P., and Pindborg, J.J.: Odontogenic tumors classification, histopathology and clinical behavior in man and domesticated animals. Cancer., 14:73-101, 1963.
3.  Bhaskar, S.N.: Adenoameloblastoma: Its histogenesis and report of 15 new cases. J. Oral Surg., 22:218-226, 1964.
4.  Philipsen, H.P., and Birn, H.: The adenomatoid odontogenic tumor. Ameloblastic adenomatoid tumor or adeno-ameloblastoma. Acta Path. Microbiol. Scandinav., 75:375-398, 1969.
5.  Chambers, K.S.: The adenoameloblastoma. Brit. J. Oral Surg., 10:310-320, 1973.
6.  Lucas, R.B.: Pathology of Oral Tumors in Children, in: Oral Pathology in the Child. International Academy of Oral Pathology, New York, 1962 pp. 59-60.
7.  Abrams, A.M., Melrose, R.J., and Howell, F.V.: Adenoameloblastoma: A clinical pathologic study of 10 new cases. Cancer, 22:175-185, 1968.
8.  Giansanti, J.S. Someren, A., and Waldron, C.A.: Odontogenic adenomatoid tumor (adenoameloblastoma). Survey of 111 cases. Oral Surg., 30:69-86, 1970.

## ODONTOGENIC TUMORS

These tumors all represent overgrowths of tooth forming tissue. Odontogenic epithelium at different stages of development has a potential to produce change in adjacent connective tissue. Classification of tumors are made on this basis. Major categories include compound odontoma, complex odontoma and ameloblastic odontoma.

## ODONTOMA

An odontoma is a benign tumor arising from mature dental structures, enamel, dentin or cementum. The compound odontoma is the commonest of these tumors, ameloblastic the least common.

The complex odontomas have poor differentiation as compared to the compound type so that calcified material with radiopacities on radiographs are seen, but there is little resemblance to a tooth. Most patients are females in 10-30 years age range. Most occur at the second and third molar region in the mandible and may be associated with an unerupted tooth (1-4).

The hard or compound odontoma has an advanced differentiation, and the calcified structure can be distinguished as teeth (1-3) (Fig. 24 a, b, c, d, e). Such tumors are classified as compound composite odontoma when they bear some resemblance to teeth (Fig. 25 a, b, c). Cementum deposition may be excessive when examined by light microscopy (3). Most occur in the upper jaw in the incisor cuspid area, and may occur between the roots of deciduous teeth. Most are diagnosed in young adults (1, 2). Multiple odontomas suggest underlying disorders such as Gardner's syndrome (Fig. 26 a, b).

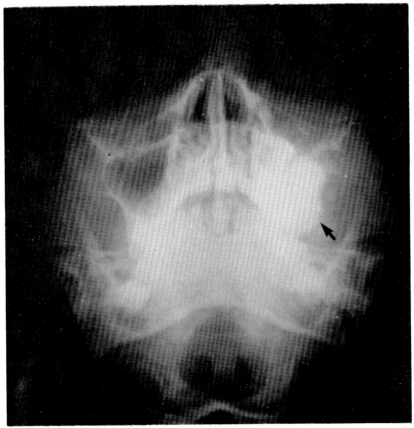

Figure 24a. 15-year-old male with history of missing teeth. A dense circumscribed bony mass with teeth, which is a compound odontoma is seen protruding into the maxilla *(arrow)*.

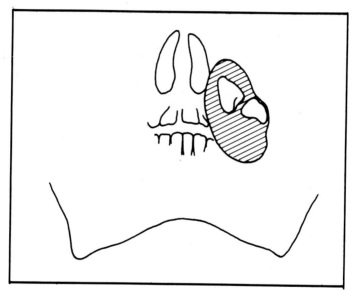

Figure 24b. Sketch.

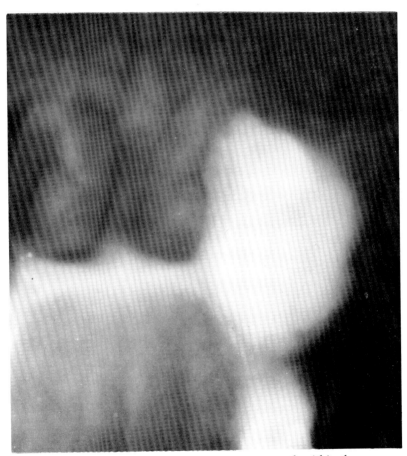

Figure 24c. Frontal laminogram demonstrates teeth within the mass.

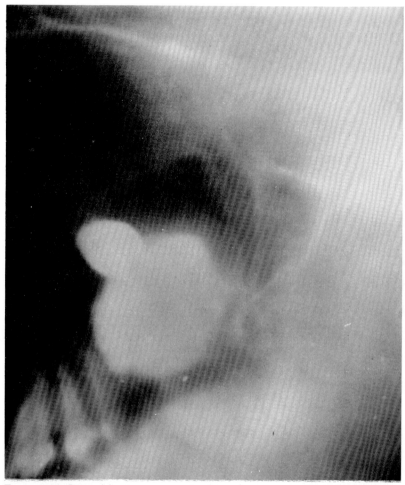

Figure 24d. Lateral laminogram again shows large mass with teeth extending into the maxillary sinus.

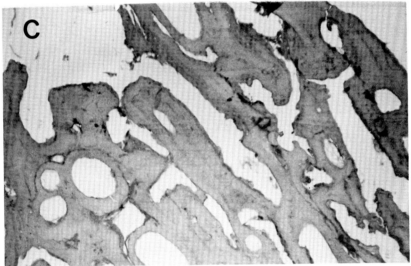

Figure 24e. A photomicrograph shows that many denticles resembling miniature malformed teeth are present (courtesy of Dr. Paul Szanto, Department of Pathology, Cook County Hospital).

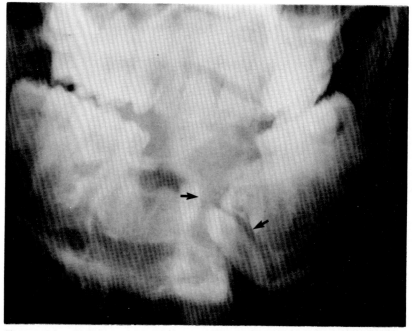

Figure 25a. Mass in the anterior mandible picked up after injury shows unerupted cuspid tooth associated with a compound composite odontoma *(arrows)*.

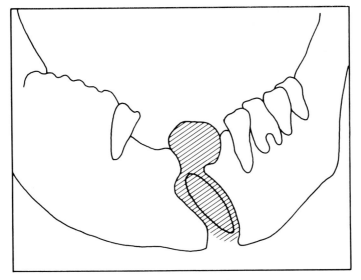

Figure 25b. Sketch.

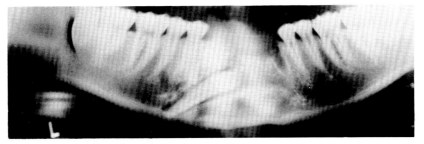

Figure 25c. Panorex shows tumor mass.

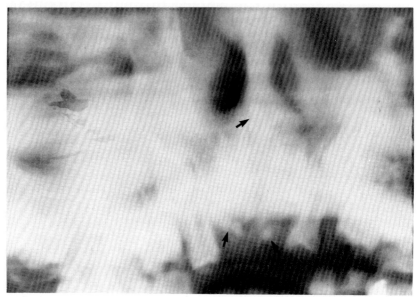

Figure 26a. Amorphous sclerotic lesions of the maxilla *(arrows);* an odontoma.
Patient was shown to have Gardner's syndrome after this diagnosis was made.

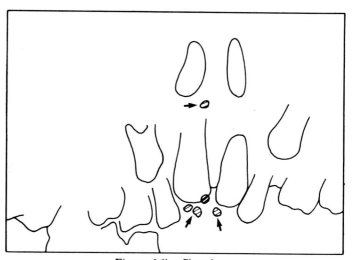

Figure 26b. Sketch.

A soft odontoma sometimes called an "ameloblastic fibroma" (1, 2, 4), is rare and may be composed of odontogenic epithelium and mesenchyme. The lesion appears like a cyst on the radiograph (Fig. 27 a, b, c) and cannot always be distinguished from other cysts or ameloblastoma. The tumor is associated frequently with unerupted teeth and may spread roots of adjacent teeth (5). Almost all occur in children (6).

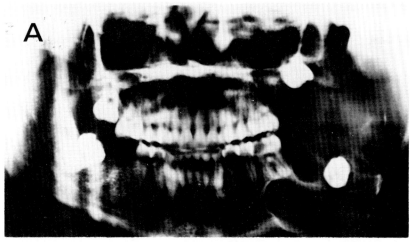

Figure 27a. Radiolucent area in the mandible with a tooth in the inferior portion. The ectopically situated molar suggests a tumor of odontogenic origin.

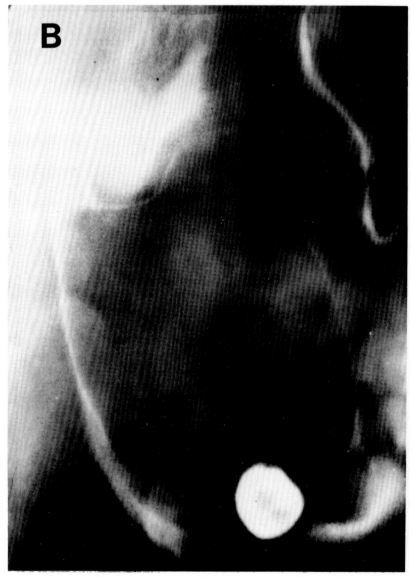

Figure 27b. Laminogram of part of the tumor shows defined walls and a tooth.

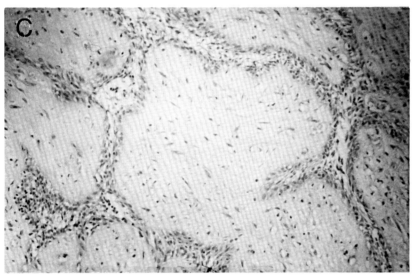

Figure 27c. Strands of a myeloblastic epithelium surrounded by and inter-
mingled with cellular fibroblastic tissue, on a photomicrograph. (Courtesy of
Dr. Paul Szanto, Department of Pathology, Cook County Hospital).

## AMELOBLASTIC ODONTOMA

Ameloblastic odontoma is a rare tumor of mixed epithelial and mesenchymal origin. There are features of both ameloblastoma and compound or complex odontoma within the tumor. In the ameloblastic odontoma, large amounts of calcified dental tissue are formed. These tend to grow slowly in either mandible or maxilla, in the premolar and molar areas and they may be expansile, destructive or behave like an odontoma (7).

On radiographs, they present as well defined radiolucent cavities unilocular or multilocular, within which are malformed tooth elements. The tumor may be encapsulated with sclerotic bone surrounding it (8, 1, 2).

On histological examination, various odontogenic tissues will be seen as well as rosette or strands of proliferating odontogenic epithelium. These tumors are usually found in children below the age of 15 years (1 and 2).

## ODONTOGENIC FIBROMA

The odontogenic fibroma is a rare odontogenic tumor of mesodermal origin (connective tissue elements) which may be seen in the maxilla or mandible. Most patients are young, between 10-29 years of age (9).

Clinically, the features are those of other jaw tumors, gradual enlargement of the jaw, with facial deformity, with no pain. Displaced teeth may be visible.

On radiographs, there is a well-defined radiolucent cyst which is not specific and may resemble an odontogenic cyst or ameloblastoma (10 and 11). The margins may be scalloped.

These tumors appear at the site of unerupted or previously erupted teeth, and are thought to be derived from the connective tissue of the follicle of the unerupted tooth (12).

## References

*Odontomas*

1. Gorlin, R.J., Chaudhry, A.P., and Pindborg, J.J.: Odontogenic tumors. Classification, histopathology and clinical behavior in man and domesticated animals. Cancer, 14:73-101, 1961.
2. Gorlin, R.J., and Goldman, H.M.: In Thoma's Oral Pathology. C.V. Mosby Co. St. Louis, 1970, 286-347, 481-515.
3. Soni, N.N., and Simpson, T.H.: Compound composite odontoma. Oral Surg., 25:556-563, 1968.

4. Jaffe, H.L.: Tumors and Tumorous Conditions of the Bone and Joint. Lee and Febiger. Philadelphia, 1961. pp. 425, 446-448.

5. Hager, R.C., Taylor, C.G., and Allen, P.M.: Ameloblastic fibroma: Report of case. J. Oral Surg., 36:66-69, 1978.

6. Novince, W.M., and Grau, W.H.: Ameloblastic fibroma. J. Oral Surg., 35:150-152, 1977.

7. Hamner, J.E., and Pizer, M.E.: Ameloblastic odontoma. Report of two cases. Amer. J. Dis. Child., 115:332-336, 1968.

8. Caruso, W., and Itkin, A.: Ameloblastic odontoma. Report of case. Oral Surg., 16:582-585, 1963.

9. Zimmerman, C., and Dahlin, D.C.: Myxomatomas tumors of the jaws. Oral Surg., 11:1069-1080, 1956.

10. Hamner, J.E., Gamble, J.W., and Gallegos, G.J.: Odontogenic fibroma. Oral Surg., 21:113-119, 1966.

11. Thompson, C., and Bolden, T.E.: Odontoma in an 11 year old boy. A case report. New York State Dent. J., 35:82-90, 1969.

12. Pincock, L.D., and Bruce, K.W.: Odontogenic fibroma. Oral Surg., 7:307-311, 1954.

# 4

# NONODONTOGENIC TUMORS

## HEMANGIOMA

Hemangioma of the oral mucosa is a common lesion; in contrast it is rare in the bone of the mandible or maxilla (1). Although hemangiomas of the jawbone appears as benign lesions, they may prove to be exceedingly hazardous, since profuse bleeding after extraction or biopsy has been a common experience, in vascular types of hemangioma (2 and 4). Palladino in a review of the literature found 31 cases of hemangioma, four of whom had a fatal outcome after extraction and seven who had severe hemorrhage after extraction or surgery (5). These tumors are composed of dilated blood vessels, fibrous tissue and large feeding vessels.

Radiographic identification may be difficult unless radiolucent defects, outlining vascular channels are seen in the plain film. Altered poorly defined density, either increased or decreased from normal is the common finding (Fig. 28 a, b) and the mental foramen may be large. Hemangiomas of the maxilla or mandible may or may not show the classical "Honeycomb" appearance. Bony spicules may radiate vertically from the center giving a sunburst effect. In general, there is neither periosteal reaction or phleboliths or other vascular calcifications seen. When teeth are involved the roots may be resorbed and the lamina dura eroded (2, 3, 6, 7). Differential diagnosis, particularly when hemangiomas are small, may vary from odontogenic tumors to mxyoma. An arteriogram is essential to exclude these lesions and identify the feeding vessels (4, 8).

Two thirds of reported tumors occurred in the body of the mandible (10). The peak incidence is in the second decade (10 and 11). Clinical findings of bleeding, swelling and a visible purplish, compressible and pulsating mass may be present.

Pericoronal oozing of blood and up and down motion of the teeth in the involved region are common symptoms (9). Asymmetry of the face may occur. Bleeding in spurts between the teeth and a spongy sensation on compression of the teeth are also described (8). In the past, treatment has centered about radiation therapy to control bleeding and shrink the tumor (2).

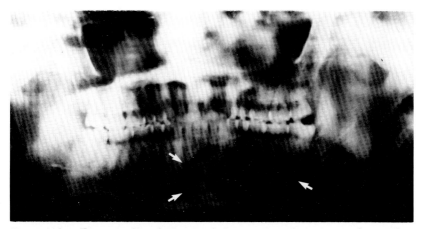

Figure 28a. Tiny specks of increased density may be seen in the midline *(arrows)* at the site of a hemangioma.

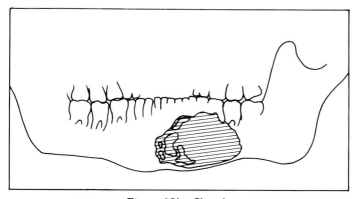

Figure 28b. Sketch.

Extensive resection of the mandible or the maxilla has proved to be necessary if bleeding could not be controlled. Ligation of one or both external carotid arteries was often necessary to control bleeding. More recently, embolization of feeding vessels with gel foam has been attempted to help control bleeding at the time of surgery (4).

## References

1. Shklar, G., and Meyer, I.: Vascular tumors of the mouth and jaws. Oral Surg., 335-358, 1965.
2. Worth, H.M.: Principles and Practice of Oral Radiologic Interpretation. Chicago Yearbook Medical Publishers, Inc. 1963, pp. 522-528.
3. Laws, I.M.: Pulsating haemangiomata of the jaws. Br. J. Oral Surg., 5:223-229, 1968.
4. Hoey, M.F., Courage, G.R., Newton, T.H., and Hoyt, W.F.: Management of vascular malformations of the mandible and maxilla: Review and report of two cases treated by embolization and surgical obliteration. J. Oral Surg., 28:696-706, 1970.
5. Gamez-Araujo, J.J., Toth, B.B., and Luna, M.A.: Central hemangioma of the mandible and maxilla: Review of a vascular lesion. Oral Surg., 37:230-238, 1974.
6. Palladino, V.S., and Danziger, A.E.: Hemangioma of the maxilla. J. Am. Dent. Assoc., 70:636-641, 1965.
7. Lund, B.A., and Dahlin, D.C.: Hemangioma of the mandible and maxilla. J. Oral Surg., 22:234-242, 1964.
8. Sherman, R.S., and Wilner, D.: The roentgen diagnosis of hemangioma of bone. Am. J. Roentgenol., 86:1146-1159, 1961.
9. Walker, D.G.: Benign non-odontogenic tumors of the jaws. J. Oral Surg., 28:39-57, 1970.
10. Stafne, E.C.: Oral Roentgenographic Diagnosis. Ed 3. Philadelphia W.B. Saunders Co., 1969, pp 198-199.
11. Thoma, K.H., and Goldman, H.M.: Oral Pathology. Ed 5. St. Louis. C.V. Mosby Co., 1960. Chap. 43-44.

## TERATOMAS

Teratomas are neoplasms of congenital origin which consist of multiple tissues foreign to the part of the body in which they arise. Although rare, the total number of cases found in children is significant in reported series (1-5). The term teratoma is used to include teratoid or dermoid tumors and epignathi. Epignathi are differentiated from other types by the presence of formed organs.

Teratomas of the face in newborns have been described (5) although teratomas originating or spreading to the maxilla are exceedingly rare (1). Teratoid cysts have linings varying from simple stratified squamous to ciliated respiratory epithelium. These may be accompanied by derivatives of entoderm, mesoderm and ectoderm. Teratoid cysts are the rarest of dermoid cysts in the head and neck (3). Teratoid tumor or teratoma in the facial area may expand facial bones with or without cortical destruction. We have seen infants in whom portions of maxillary and mandible were so expanded that they were no longer visible (Fig. 29 a, b, c, d). Despite this, the growth of the tumor was slow and the tumor was benign histologically. There were no calcifications present that are ordinarily associated with teratoma. Since this lesion was present at birth, it conceivably represents a developmental error rather than being a true tumor.

## References

1. Partlow, W.F. and Taybi, H.: Teratomas in infants and children. Am. J. Roentgen. 112:115-166, 1971.
2. Willis, R.A.: The pathology of tumors of children. Charles C. Thomas Publishers, Springfield, Illinois. 1962, pp. 76-92.
3. Batsakis, J.G.: Tumors of the head and neck. Williams and Wilkins, Boston, 1974, 155-161.
4. Ariel, I.M. and Pack, G.T.: Cancer and allied disease in infancy and childhood. Little Brown and Co. Boston, 1959, 249-273.
5. Tefft, M., Vawter, G. and Neuhauser, E.B.D.: Unusual facial tumors in the newborn. Am. J. Roentgen. 95:32-40, 1965.
6. Dicke, T.E. and Gates, G.A.: Malignant teratoma of the paranasal sinuses. Arch Otolaryng. 91:391-394, 1970.
7. Patchefsky, A., Sundmaker, W. and Marden, P.A.: Malignant teratoma of the ethmoid sinus. Cancer. 21:714-721, 1968.
8. Sollee, A.N.: Nasopharyngeal teratoma. Arch Otolaryng. 82:49-52, 1965.

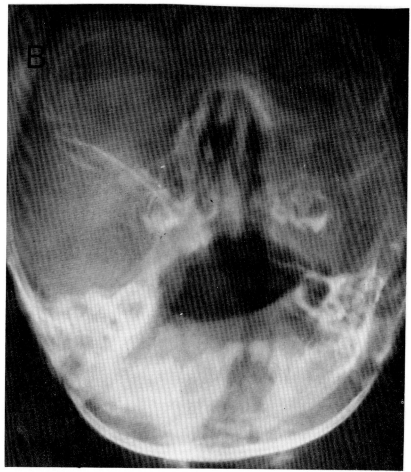

Figure 29a. A cystic mass over the right zygoma was noted at birth. Films show an extensive mass occupying maxilla and ramus of the mandible, which proved to be a benign teratoid cyst.

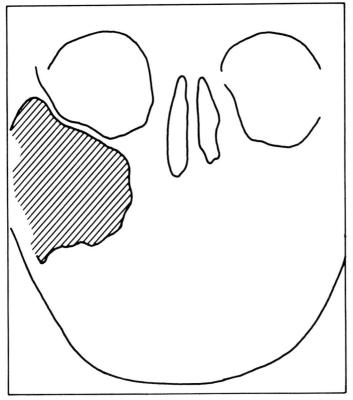

Figure 29b. Sketch.

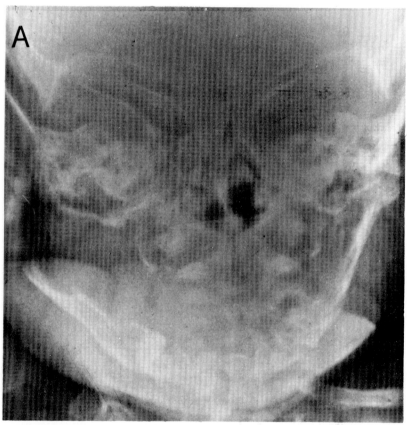

Figure 29c.  View of the mandible shows erosion by tumor mass.

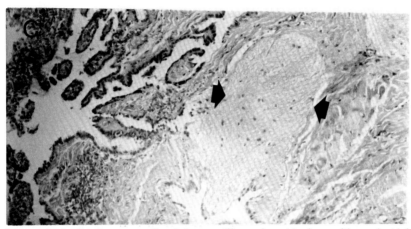

Figure 29d. Cystic spaces lined by papillary choroid plexus like cuboidal epithelium. There are alternating bands of connective tissue and neuroglial tissue *(arrows)* in the cyst wall. (Courtesy of Dr. Paul Szanto, Department of Pathology, Cook County Hospital).

Teratomas of the face, like teratomas elsewhere, present a spectrum according to the rate of growth and differentiation of the tumor. Tumors may be cystic, solid or a combination of both and may arise from or invade the maxilla. Figure 30 a, b, c, d shows a 16-year-old patient in whom a malignant teratoma arose in the ethmoid sinus, extended to maxillary antrum, nasal cavity and invaded the adjacent bone. It is exceedingly rare in this location in a young patient and there are few instances in adults (6, 7). Radiographically, it cannot be distinguished from other maxillary and nasal tumors except for the presence of bone destruction.

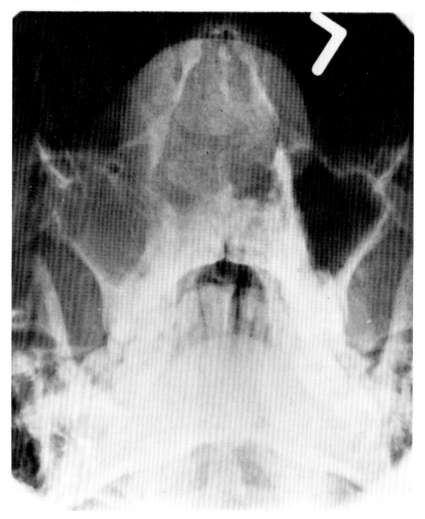

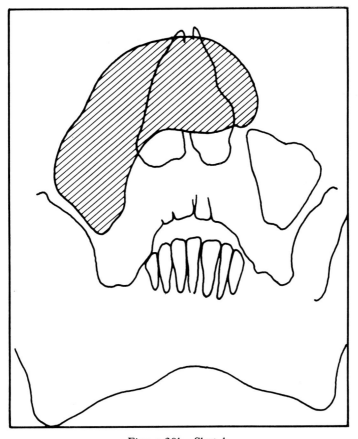

Figure 30b. Sketch.

←

Figure 30a. A 16-year-old male presented with nasal congestion and a soft
tissue mass extending from nose. Facial bone views show a mass in the
ethmoids, right maxillary antrum and nose. Tumor recurred twice, at 3 months
and one year post operatively.

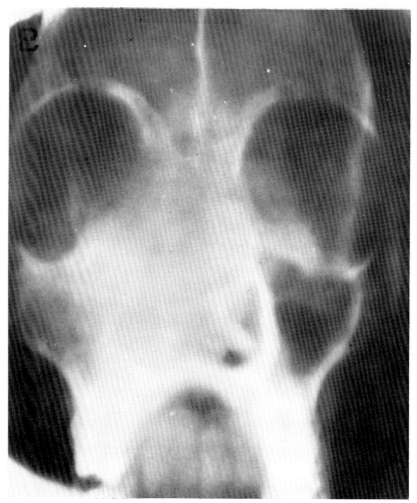

Figure 30c. Frontal laminogram shows large destructive tumor. Histology was malignant teratoma.

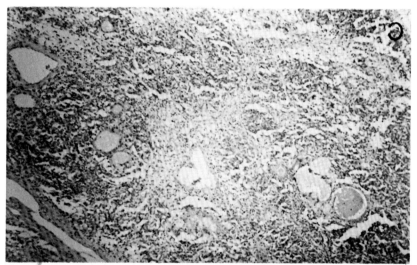

Figure 30d. Malignant teratoma with neuroblastic differentiation. Primary tumor is a highly cellular tumor composed chiefly of small neuroblast like primitive cells with focal glandular differentiation. (Courtesy of Dr. Paul Szanto, Department of Pathology, Cook County Hospital).

Teratomas of the nasopharynx arise from midline, are generally present at birth, and most are dermoid cysts (8). Teratomas may spread to the maxillae but rarely do so. A teratoid mass in the neck may interfere with the formation or the hard and soft palate and may encroach on and deform the mandible (Fig. 31, a, b).

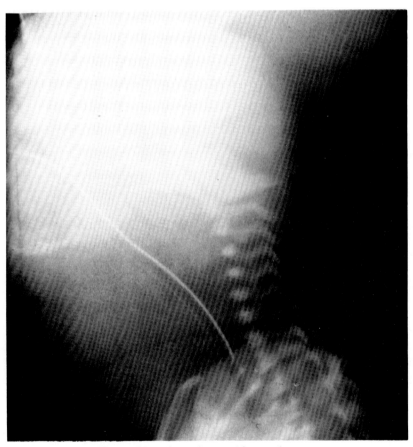

Figure 31a. A newborn with a neck mass.

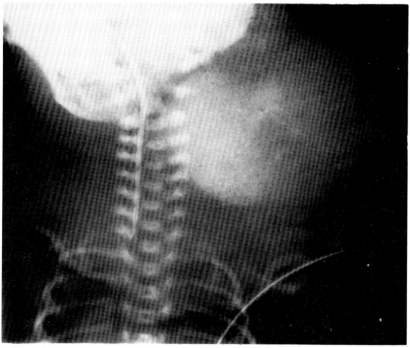

Figure 31b. Faint calcifications are present within the mass which is deforming the mandible. The airway is compressed by the tumor.

## MELANOTIC NEUROECTODERMAL TUMORS

Among tumors in infancy which present as a jaw bone mass is melanotic neuroectodermal tumor of infancy (Fig. 1). This is a benign tumor of neural crest origin, seen before the age of 1 year, most commonly in the maxilla, and in females (1 and 6). About 15% of these tumors recur locally, and are very rarely malignant (7). The name melanotic prognoma is based on Stowen's opinion that these tumors represent an atavism of sensory neuroectodermal development (1, 3 and 5). The tumor is frequently associated with dental structures, sometime abnormally developed tooth buds (1). Other names such as melanotic ameloblastomas have been suggested by those who believe there is an odontogenic origin (1 and 2). A report of a case with elevated urinary excretion of vanilmandelic acid suggests that the tumor is of neural crest origin (6). Also elevated VMA levels in association with recurrent lesions is supporting evidence of neural crest origin (8).

On radiographs, displacement of teeth and destruction of alveolar bone may be seen. Most lesions have been described in the anterior maxilla (6) (Fig. 32).

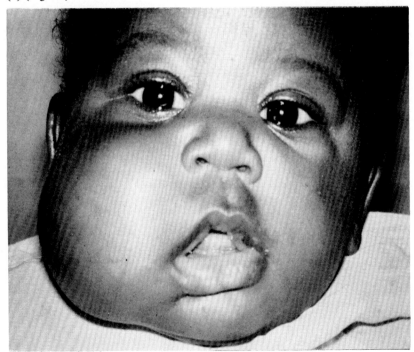

Figure 32. Frontal view of the face depicting a large soft tumor mass of the right cheek, epicanthal folds, flat nasal bridge and mild hypertelorism. (Courtesy of Dr. Joanna Seibert, Arkansas Children's Hospital.)

## References

1. Tieke, R.W., and Bernier, J.L.: Melanotic ameloblastoma. Oral Surg., 9:1197-1209, 1956.
2. Lurie, H.I.: Congenital melanocarcinoma, melanotic adamantinoma, retinal anlage tumor, progonoma and pigmented epulis of infancy. Cancer, 14:1090-1108, 1961.
3. Medenis, R., Slaughter, D.P., and Barber, T.K.: Melanotic progonoma in childhood. Pediatrics, 29:600-604, 1962.
4. Kerr, D.A., and Weiss, A.W.: Pigmented ameloblastoma of the mandible: Report of a case. Oral Surg., 16:1339-1343, 1963.
5. Kerr, D.A., and Pullon, P.A.: A study of the pigmented tumors of jaws of infants (Melanotic ameloblastoma, retinal anlage tumor, progonoma). Oral Surg., 18:759-772, 1964.
6. Borello, E.D., and Gorlin, R.J.: Melanotic neuroectodermal tumor of infancy: A neoplasm of neural crest origin. Cancer, 19:196-206, 1966.
7. Block, J.C., Waite, D.E., Dehner, L.P., Leonard, A.S., Ogle, R.G., and Gatto, D.J.: Pigmented neuroectodermal tumor of infancy. Oral Surg., 49:279-285, 1980.
8. Brekke, J.H., and Gorlin, R.J.: Melanotic neuroectodermal tumor of infancy. J. Oral Surg., 33:858-865, 1975.

# 5

## MALIGNANT TUMORS OF JAW BONE

### OSTEOGENIC SARCOMA

Osteogenic sarcoma occurs mainly between 10-25 years of age, is twice as frequent in males and rare in jaws. Clinically, the presentation, is that of pain, swelling, facial asymmetry. The tumor is subdivided into osteoblastic and osteoclastic forms. On radiographs, the osteoblastic type is radiopaque (Fig. 33 a, b), produces a sun-ray appearance in a small percentage of cases and expands the cortical plates while the osteolytic type produces irregular radiolucency. Histologically, these are derived from multipotential cells so that in osteoblastic type one sees osteoblasts, chondrocytes and spindle cells. In the osteolytic form, bone destruction is seen as well as osteoblasts and spindle cells. Despite treatment with radical surgery, the prognosis is very poor, but slightly better for the mandible than long bones. Recurrence occurs more often in the mandible; metastasis usually go to the lung via the lung vessels (1, 2). Osteogenic sarcoma in irradiated bones occurs after an irradiation dosage over 3,000 rad; there may be microscopic or radiographic evidence of a benign primary lesion.

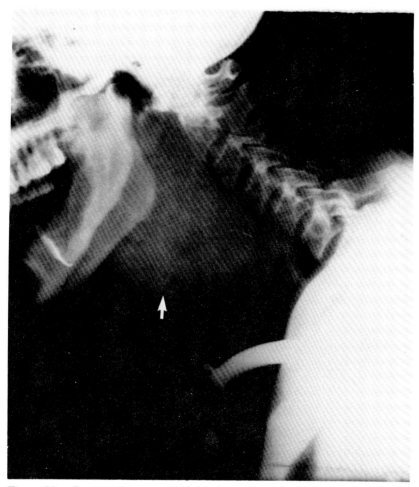

Figure 33a. Osteogenic sarcoma arising from ramus and body of the mandible with a large calcified mass *(arrow)*. (Courtesy of Dr. G. Espinosa, Westside V.A. Hospital, Chicago).

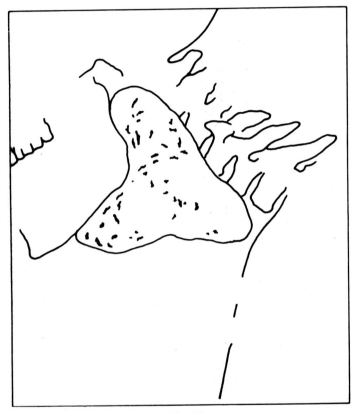

Figure 33b. Sketch.

## CHONDROSARCOMA

Chondrosarcoma compared to osteogenic sarcoma is less common, appears at a later age and has a slower course. It is classified as primary (from vestigial rest of cartilage) or secondary (from pre-existing benign cartilagenous tumors), the secondary being more common, although both are rare. It originates from areas which are preformed in cartilage. The tumor occurs equally in both sexes; in adults 30 to 50 years of age. Clinically, like a chondroma, it presents with a painless expanding lesion causing resorption and loosening of the teeth. The radiographic picture is not definitive and looks like a chondroma. There may be radiolucent defects with speckled calcifications (3). On histological examination, there is considerable variation in different areas. Many cells have plump nuclei or two such nuclei; giant cartilage cells with clumped chromatin present; active growth resides in the undifferentiated peripheral cells (3, 4). The prognosis is poor but better than osteogenic sarcoma. Tumors which occur in the jaw have a poorer prognosis than those which occur in the long bones; metastasis go to the lungs (Fig. 34 a, b).

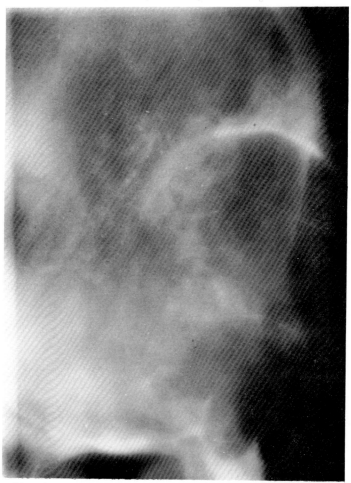

Figure 34a. Anteroposterior tomogram of the left maxilla demonstrates a mass density in the left maxilla with destruction of the floor of the orbit and extension to the ethmoidal and frontal sinus and extension across the midline to the right maxilla. This was a chondrosarcoma of the left maxillary sinus region.

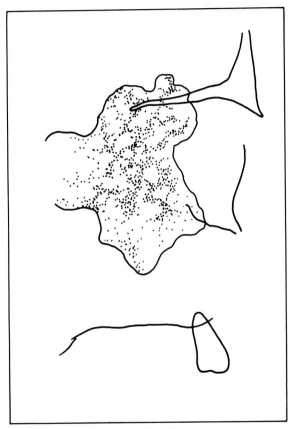

Figure 34b. Sketch.

## SQUAMOUS CELL CARCINOMA

This is the most common malignancy in the oral cavity (2). Intraosseous carcinoma of the jaws may arise from epithelial remnants or secondary to long standing chronic inflammation involving squamous epithelium (Fig. 35 a, b). These tumors are rare, occur in middle age and present as a radiolucent moth eaten appearance on radiographs (Fig. 36 a, b, c).

Carcinoma has been described arising from the walls of cysts (5). Gardner reviewed the literature and found 25 well documented cases of squamous cell carcinoma which had its origin in an odontogenic cyst (6). Among these, the median age was 57. Clinical findings included rapid increase in jaw size, failure of the extraction site to heal, displacement of teeth and appearance of a flat or papilliferous mass attached to the base at the time of enucleation. On radiographs the radiolucencies in the jaw had ill defined jagged borders with resorption of the roots of adjacent teeth (6).

Newer techniques such as CAT scans are useful in identifying the extent of the tumor (Fig. 37 a, b).

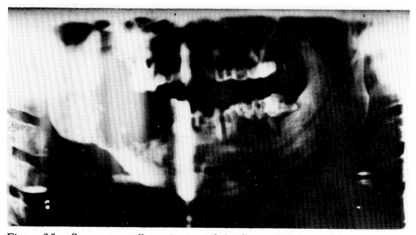

Figure 35a. Squamous cell carcinoma of the floor of the mouth with invasion and destruction of the right mandible.

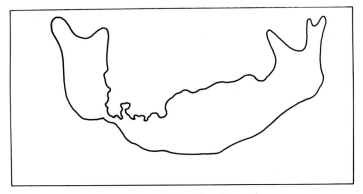

Figure 35b. Sketch.

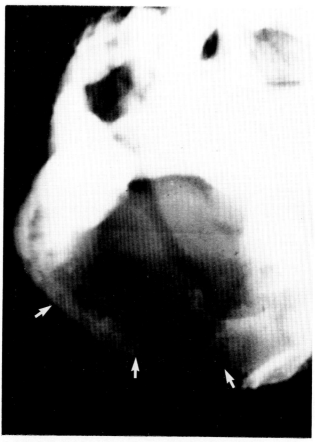

Figure 36a. Deeply erosive squamous cell carcinoma. Mandible is expanded, partially destroyed and shows evidence of extensive invasion.

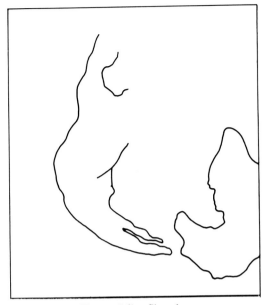

Figure 36b. Sketch.

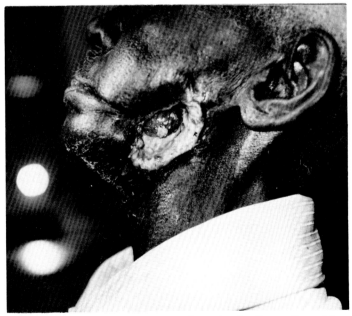

Figure 36c. Patient showing massive ulceration by the malignant tumor.

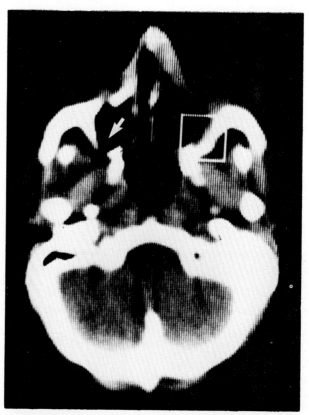

Figure 37a. Transverse axial C.T. showing destruction of the anteromedial wall of the right maxillary antrum by squamous cell carcinoma of the right maxillary sinus *(arrow)*.

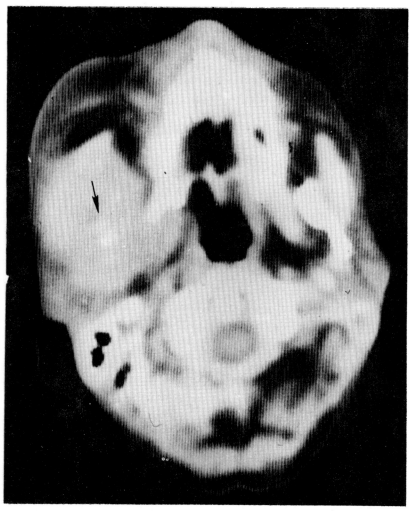

Figure 37b. Axial C.T. scan demonstrates lobulated, well defined mass in the right parotid region showing central calcification *(arrow)*, with extension to the right ramus of the mandible.

## References

1.   Wood, N., Goaz, P.W., and Stuteville, O.H.: Differential Diagnosis of Oral Lesions. C.V. Mosby and Co. 381-396, 1975.
2.   Baker, C.G., and Tishler, J.M.: "Malignant disease of the jaws." J. Can. Assoc. Radiol., 28:129-141, 1977.
3.   Nortje, C.J., Farman, A.G., Grotepass, F.W., and Van Zyl, J.A.: Chondro-sarcoma of the mandibular condyle: Report of a case with special reference of radiographic features. Br. J. Oral Surg., 14:101-111, 1976.
4.   Sato, K., Nukaga, H., and Horikoshi, T.: Chondrosarcoma of the jaws and facial skeleton: A review of the Japanese literature. J. Oral Surg., 35:892-897, 1977.
5.   Kay, L.W., and Kramer, I.R.H.: Squamous cell carcinoma arising in a dental cyst. Oral Surg., 15:970-979, 1962.
6.   Gardner, A.F.: The odontogenic cyst as a potential carcinoma: A clinico-pathologic appraisal. J. Am. Dent. Assoc., 78:746-755, 1969.

## BURKITT'S LYMPHOMA

A sarcoma of the jaws was first described by Christiansen in 1938 (1), but brought to general attention by Burkitt in 1958 (2) when he described 38 children in Uganda with this tumor. The most common site he described was in the maxilla. The tumor grew rapidly with early involvement of the maxilla. Loosening of the teeth was an early sign, with the tumor showing rapid growth and distortion as well as destruction of tissues in its path. Adrenal, kidney and liver metastases were commonly reported (2). In the 1960's, chemo-therapy utilizing methotrezate and cyclophosphamid had been described as successful in providing remissions in most cases (3).

Lymphomas of childhood which histologically resemble Burkitt's tumor occur in the United States but rarely involve the jaw bones (4-7). There have been suggestions that the tumor is virus related, either to the Epstein-Barr virus or the reovirus (8).

The very first sign are tiny areas of bone destruction in the jaws best seen near erosions of the lamina dura.

The earliest radiographic signs consist of small areas of destruction in the bone around the roots of teeth usually molars (Fig. 38 a, b), (Fig. 39 a, b). These foci increase in size rapidly, coalesce and break through the alveolar margin and inner jaw surface (Fig. 40 a, b). Markedly destroyed bone within which a few strands of bone lie may suggest osteomyelitis with sequestra formation (9-12).

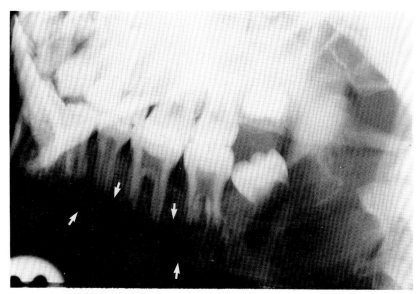

Figure 38a. Very early phase of Burkitt's with lucencies around roots of molar teeth *(arrows)*. (Courtesy of Dr. W.P. Cockshott, McMaster Univ. Med. Center., Hamilton, Ontario, Canada).

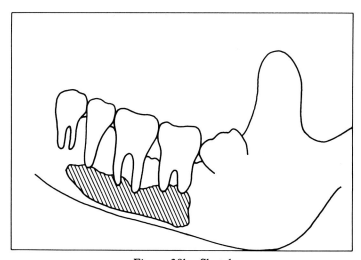

Figure 38b. Sketch.

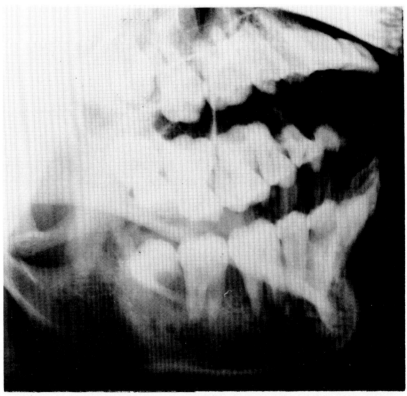

Figure 39a. An early phase of Burkitt's lymphoma showing destruction of the bone around roots of molars. (Courtesy of Dr. W.P. Cockshott, McMaster Univ. Med. Center, Hamilton, Ontario, Canada.)

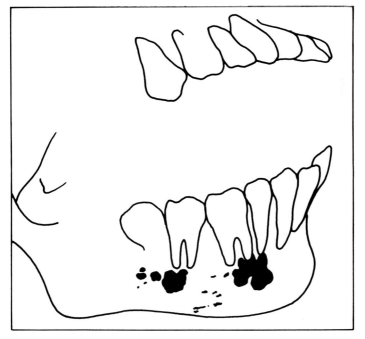

Figure 39b. Sketch.

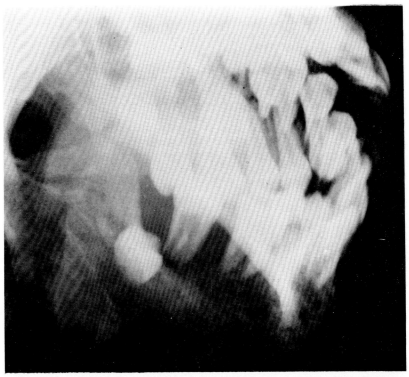

Figure 40a. Burkitt's lymphoma with early erosive bone destruction. (Courtesy of Dr. W.P. Cockshott, McMaster Univ. Med. Center, Hamilton, Ontario, Canada.)

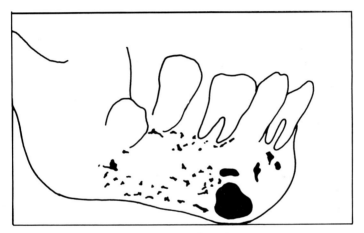

Figure 40b. Sketch.

Teeth will become embedded in the tumor as the sockets are destroyed; as the mass progresses teeth are forced upwards and fall out (Fig. 41 a, b). Maxillary tumors invade the sinuses, (Fig. 42 a, b), sphenoid wings and nasal passage (12). Infiltration through the outer mandibular border occurs more slowly and is accompanied by periosteal reaction (11, 12).

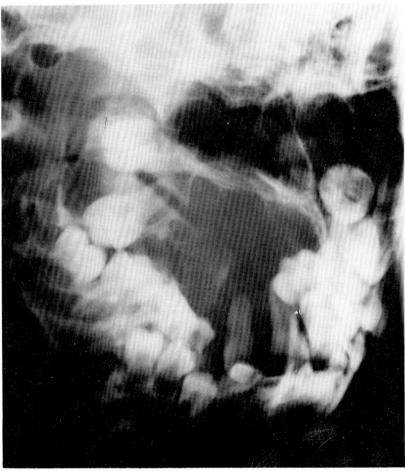

Figure 41a. Large mass distorting teeth in a patient with Burkitt's lymphoma. (Courtesy of Dr. W.P. Cockshott, McMaster Univ. Med. Center, Hamilton, Ontario, Canada.)

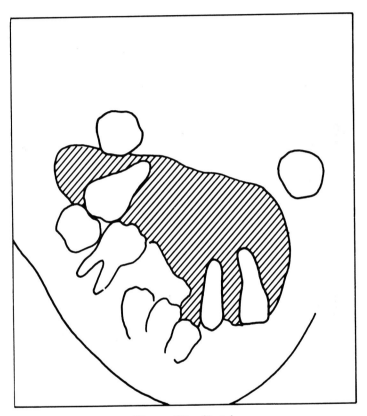

Figure 41b. Sketch.

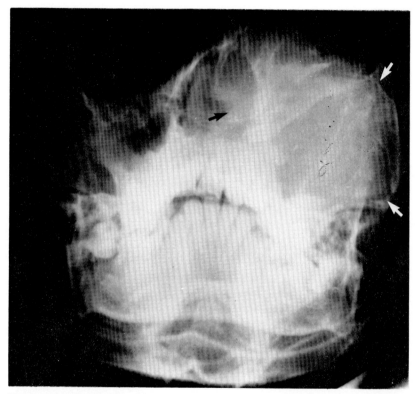

Figure 42a. Large mass of Burkitt's lymphoma invading the antrum *(arrows)*.
(Courtesy of Dr. W.P. Cockshott, McMaster Univ. Med. Center, Hamilton,
Ontario, Canada.)

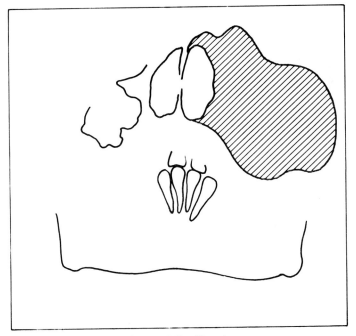

Figure 42b.  Sketch.

### References

1. Christiansen, G.W.: J. Am. Dent. Assoc., 25:725, 1938.
2. Burkitt, D.: A sarcoma involving the jaws in African children. Br. J. Surg., 46:218-223, 1958.
3. Burkitt, D.: The African lymphoma. Preliminary observations on response to therapy. Cancer, 18:399-410, 1965.
4. O'Conor, E.T., Rappaport, H., and Smith, E.B.: Childhood lymphoma resembling "Burkitt tumor" in the United States. Cancer, 18:411-417, 1965.
5. Alford, B.A., Cocci, P.R., and L'Heureux, P.R.: Roentgenographic features of American Burkitt's lymphoma. Radiology, 124:763-770, 1977.
6. Davidson, J.W., and Renouf, J.H.P.: Radiographic findings in "Burkitt type" lymphoma. J. Can. Assoc. Radiol., 19:121-125, 1968.
7. Dunnick, N.R., Reaman, G.H., Head, G.L., Shawker, T.H., and Ziegler, J.L.: Radiographic manifestations of Burkitt's lymphoma in American patients. Am. J. Roentgenol., 132:1-6, 1979.
8. Whittaker, L.R.: Burkitt's lymphoma. Clin. Radiol., 24:339-346, 1973.
9. Davies, A.G.: Cancer in East Africa. Tropical Radiology. H. Middlemiss, ed. London, William Heinemann, 1961, pp. 256-267.
10. Cockshott, P.: Cancer in West Africa. Tropical Radiology. H. Middlemiss, ed. London, William Heinemann, 1961, pp. 246-255.
11. Davies, A.G.M., and Davies, J.N.P.: Tumors of the jaw in Uganda Africans. Act. Un. Int. Cancer, 16:1320-1324, 1960.
12. Cockshott, W.P.: Radiological aspects of Burkitt's tumor. Br. J. Radiol., 38:172-180, 1965.

# 6

## FIBRO-OSSEOUS JAW BONE LESIONS

The fibro-osseous lesions of the jawbone are classified as fibrous dysplasia or ossifying fibroma. They represent the most prevalent maxillary tumor masses seen in children and young adults. The clinical presentation is, generally, that of facial deformity. The tumor will feel hard and bony on palpation (1). Although large tumors may involve the mandible without restricting jaw motion, when the maxilla is involved growth may proceed in a cranial direction displacing or invading the orbit, with expansion into the nasal passages occuring as well. Teeth may be displaced, particularly the first and second molars (2).

Fibrous dysplasia has more commonly been reported in females, and in the maxilla, rather than the mandible (3). The lesions may be monostotic, polyostotic, alone, or in association with Albright's syndrome. The radiographic features vary from well circumscribed to poorly defined ossifying lesions (1). In Houston's series, dense sclerotic lesions were seen in the maxilla, while those in the mandible were radiolucent, multilocular and osteolytic (4). The radiological appearance may be that of a well circumscribed, centrally placed maxillary expanding lesion (Fig. 43 a, b, c) or on the other hand may show a homogeneous density or ground glass appearance (Fig. 44).

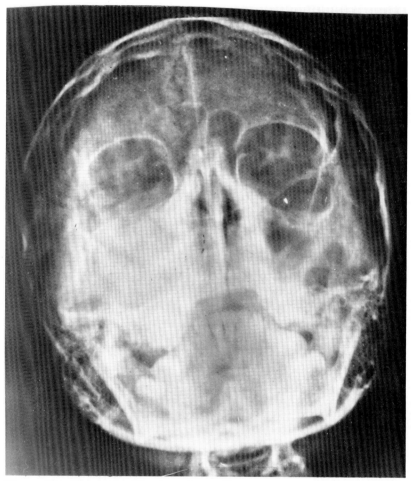

Figure 43a. Dense opacification of maxillary antrum on Water's view with destruction of medial and posterior walls of the sinus.

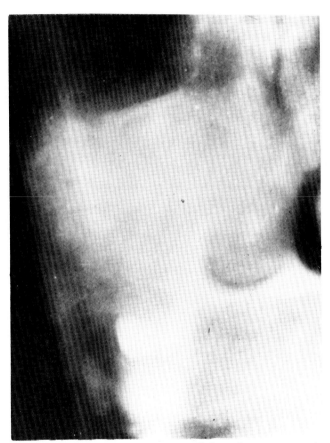

Figure 43b. Laminogram demonstrates wall loss due to expansion of the mass, proven to be fibrous dysplasia.

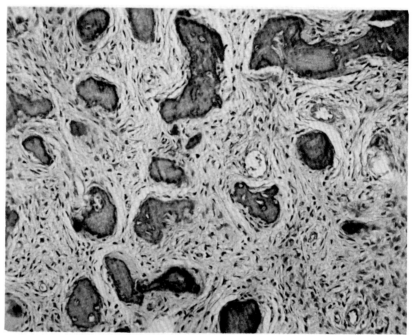

Figure 43c. Small islands of metaplastic bone amidst cellular fibroblastic tissue. (Courtesy of Dr. Paul Szanto, Department of Pathology, Cook County Hospital.)

## MONOSTOTIC FIBROUS DYSPLASIA

The age at which this is seen in the jaws tends to be in the early twenties (7) although fibrous dysplasia has been reported from 7-80 years of age (3). The lesion, although slow growing, may show growth spurts until skeletal maturation occurs (8). The fact that the majority of cases are seen in the maxilla (3), has been explained by the rapid growth of the maxilla during puberty, which is also at a period of peak incidence of fibrous dysplasia. The sex distribution favors women (4, 9 and 7).

The radiographic appearance in the maxilla may vary from expanding, dense, or sclerotic, to "ground glass." Bone formation is due to osteoblastic activity. The stippled or granular appearance is a result of bone replacement of fibrous tissue and abnormally formed osseous tissue. The histological pattern ranges from irregular bone trabeculae, woven bone, collagen formation and lamellar bone formation. Cranio-facial fibrous dysplasia show a greater proportion of bone to fibrous tissue and a tendency towards lamellar bone formation (Fig. 4-6). According to Sherman and Glauser's radiographic classification, the type most often seen in the maxilla is that with diffuse uniform sclerosis which follows the anatomical shape of bone, while enlarging it (2). Fibrous dysplasia is described as unilateral in the maxilla extending from the canine teeth to the tuberosity. As it grows, it can involve the zygomatic process, the sinus walls, the nasal cavity or floor of the orbit (8, 13) (Fig. 43 a, b). Antral and orbital encroachment are common (6).

In the mandible, lesions are more likely to be radiolucent, multiloculated and osteolytic (4), which suggests that the pathology is primarily fibrous tissue (5). The body of the mandible, body of the bone, and nontooth bearing areas are commonly involved (2, 6) (Fig. 44 a, b).

Deposits in the mandible are often oval and expansile, (12). In the mandible, the lesion may either be sclerotic or translucent with trabeculation or loculation giving a multilocular appearance (14). This is due to eroding of the original cortex of bone by the expanding lesion with distension of new cortex leaving bony ridges on the inner surface (9).

In fibrous dysplasia, connective tissue variably replace the spongiosa forming osteogenic connective tissue. This osteoid tissue grows into the marrow space and causes resorption of bony trabeculae. The presence of osteoid imparts a ground glass appearance (5). Cartilage interspersement may give a "smoke" like appearance (9). Cranio-facial lesions tend to be more osseous than elsewhere in the bony skeleton (6).

In fibrous dysplasia, there is no periosteal new bone present, which helps to distinguish it from osteomyelitis (15).

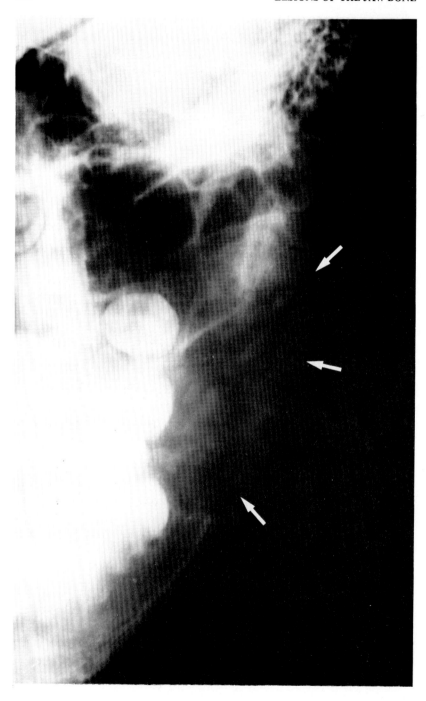

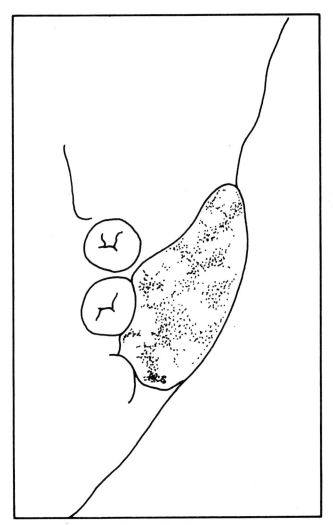

Figure 44b. Sketch.

←

Figure 44a. Groundglass appearance of fibrous dysplasia of the mandible *(arrows)*.

## POLYOSTOTIC FIBROUS DYSPLASIA

When fibrous dysplasia involves several bones and is associated with precocious puberty and areas of skin pigmentation, it is known as Albright's syndrome. The basic features include widespread skeletal changes of fibrous dysplasia, "Cafe-au-lait" pigmentation, and an endocrine disorder with sexual precocity and thyroid malfunction. Serum alkaline phosphatase may be elevated (16, 17). Synonyms for this syndrome include polyostotic fibrosa, fibrocystic disease of bone, osteofibrous deformans juveniles, polyostotic skeletal cystofibromatosis, osteitis fibroma disseminata. Reported cases have an age range of birth to 56 years (14); the majority are young women. It is a disease characterized by replacement of the marrow by fibrous tissue containing abnormal fibrous bony spicules (Fig. 45 a, b, c). The most frequent sites of involvement are the long bones and the pelvic bone (Fig. 46).

Lesions in the femur frequently are seen at the neck or intertrochanteric area. There are fusiform expansile lesions centrally translucent or ground glass. Most occur in the diaphysis of the long bone and bowing may be present. The rim may be sclerotic or poorly defined (Fig. 7), the process extending along the length of the diaphysis (11). In the ileum, the most common location is above the acetabulum. In patients in whom the ileum is involved, it may be expected that a femur will also be involved (14). Polyostotic fibrous dysplasia usually affects one side of the body. Increased density of the base of the skull was felt to be diagnostic by Harris in a series of 20 cases (11).

Radiographic features are usually cyst-like areas of translucency with coarsened trabeculae, expansion of bone, thinning of the cortex and deformity in long standing cases.

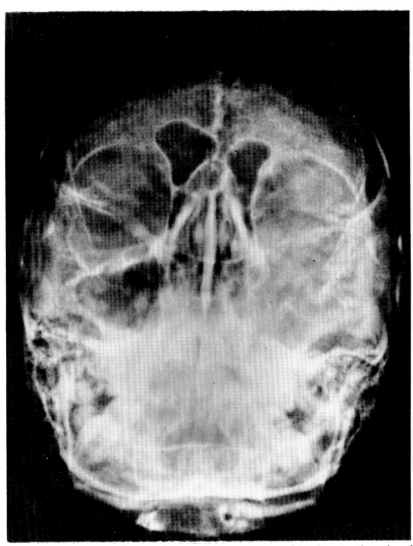

Figure 45a. 10-year-old female with 1 year history of back pain, 6 weeks of left infraorbital swelling and opacification left maxillary antrum with orbital floor destruction.

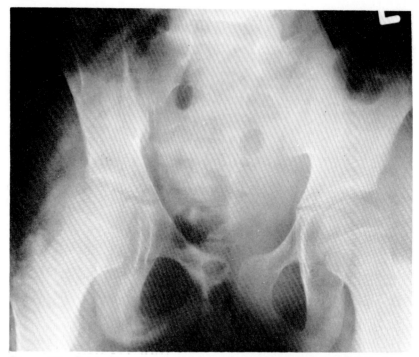

Figure 45b. Pelvis films show reticular trabecular pattern in the right ischium.

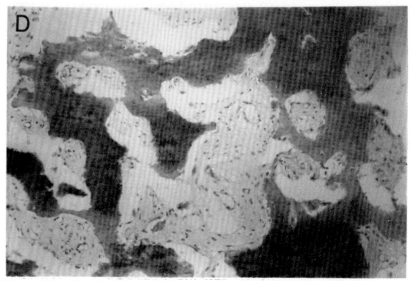

Figure 45c. The histology of a biopsy shows trabecules of immature woven bone devoid of osteoblastic rims intermingling with loose connective tissue.

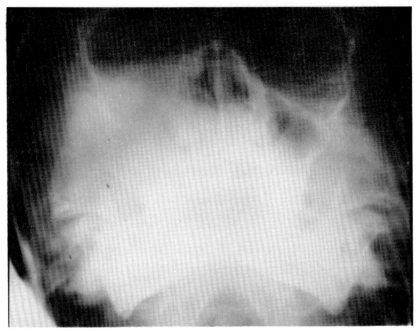

Figure 46. Opacification in an ossifying fibroma of the right maxillary sinus.

## OSSIFYING FIBROMA

Ossifying fibroma is a monostotic lesion limited to the membranous bones, generally seen in the jaw bones, and occurring during childhood (18, 19). This is a benign tumor of fibrous origin which may be locally invasive. The maxilla is a slightly more common site than the mandible and there is a female predominance (9). Fibromas of the maxillary antrum are very rare (20) and difficult to distinguish from fibrous dysplasia both clinically and radiographically (Fig. 7). The shape is said to be oval or spherical, the tumor destructive early in its course, and expansile (21). The patient presents for painless swelling of the cheek or jaw. On physical examination, there is a hard non-tender mass; bulging of the palate may be seen. On radiographs, a homogeneous opacification of the antrum with expansion will be present (Fig. 46). Histologically, the tumors are composed of fibrous connective tissue and osseous tissue, some of which is atypical bone formed by metaplasia (22). The lesion tends to have a predominant osseous element so that the radiographic appearance is ground glass or opaque (9) (Fig. 47 a, b, c, d).

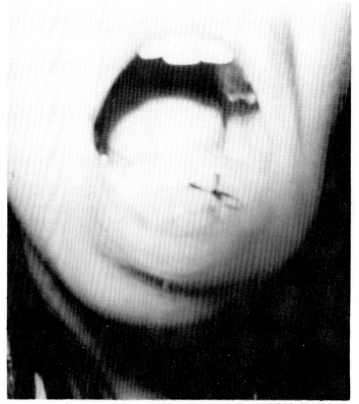

Figure 47a. A 15-year-old Mexican girl presents with recurring mass.

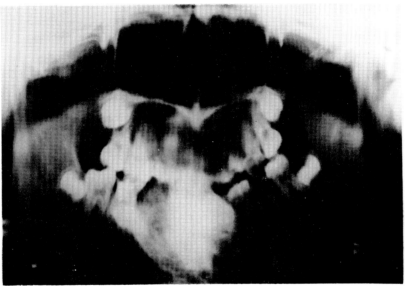

Figure 47b. Panorex shows a dense trabecular well circumscribed tumor of the mandible.

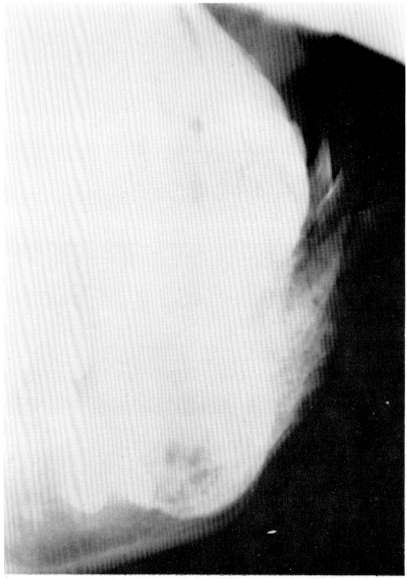

Figure 47c. Oblique view demonstrate coarse trabecular pattern.

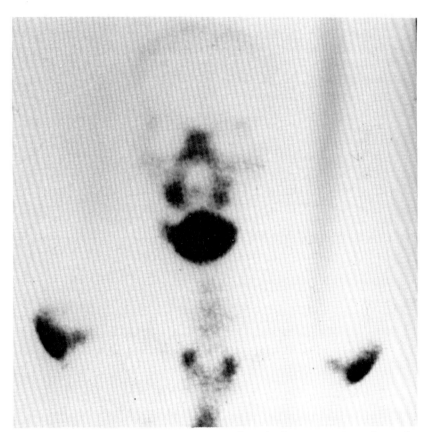

Figure 47d. On Technitium scan an area of markedly increased uptake at the tumor site was identified.

## References

1. Smith, I., and Schmanan, A.: Benign fibrous-osseous lesions of the mandible and maxilla: Clinical features. S. Afr. Med. J., 1423-1428, 1970.
2. Berger, A., and Jaffe, H.L.: Fibrous (fibro-osseous) dysplasia of jaw bones, J. Oral Surg., 11:3-17, 1953.
3. Dahlgren, S.E., Lind, P.O., Lindbom, A., and Martensson, G.: Fibrous dysplasia of jaw bones: A clinical roentgenographic and histopathologic study. Acta OtoLaryngol., 68:257-270, 1969.
4. Houston, W.O.: Fibrous dysplasia of maxilla and mandible: Clinicopathologic study and comparison of facial bone lesions with lesions affecting general skeleton. J. Oral Surg., 23:17-39, 1965.
5. Lewin, M.L.: Nonmalignant maxillofacial tumors in children: Plast. Reconstr. Surg., 38;186-196, 1966.
6. Waldron, C.A., and Giansanti, J.S.: Benign fibro-osseous lesions of the jaws: A clinical-radiologic-histologic review of sixty-five cases, Part 1. Fibrous dysplasia of the jaws. Oral Surg., 35:190-201, 1973.
7. Henry, A.: Monostotic fibrous dysplasia. JBJS, 44B:300-306, 1969.
8. Khosla, V.M., and Korobkin, M.: Monostotic fibrous dysplasia of the jaw: Report of three cases. J. Oral Surg., 29:507-513, 1971.
9. Jaffe, H.L.: Tumors and Tumorous Conditions of the Bone and Joint. Lee and Febiger. Philadelphia, 1961, pp. 117-142.
10. Waldron, C.A.: Fibro-osseous lesions of the jaws. J. Oral Surg., 28:58-64, 1970.
11. Harris, W.H., Dudley, R.H., and Barry, R.J.: The natural history of fibrous dysplasia. JBJS, 44A:207-233, 1962.
12. Sherman, R.S., and Glauser, O.J.: Radiological identification of fibrous dysplasia of the jaws. Radiology, 71:553-558, 1958.
13. Cangiano, R., Stratigos, G.T., and Williams, F.A.: Clinical and radiographic manifestations of fibro-osseous lesions of the jaws: Report of five cases. J. Oral Surg., 29:872-881, 1971.
14. Gibson, M.J., and Middlemiss, J.H.: Fibrous dysplasia of bone. Br. J. Radiol., 44:1-13, 1971.
15. Worth, H.M., and Stoneman, D.W.: Osteomyelitis, malignant disease and fibrous dysplasia. Some radiologic similarities and differences. Dent. Radiogr. Photogr., 50:1-8, 12, 1977.
16. Stewart, M.J., Gilmer, W.S., and Edmonson, A.S.: Fibrous dysplasia of bone. JBJS, 44B:302-318, 1962.
17. Church, L.E.: Polyostotic fibrous dysplasia of bone. Oral Surg., 11:184-196, 1958.
18. Knabe, G.W.: Fibrous dysplasia of the mandible. Oral Surg., 10:285-295, 1957.

19. Grewal, B.S., Nirola, A., and Verma, S.K.: Maxillary fibroma. Oral Surg., 25:175-178, 1968.
20. Sherman, R.S., and Sternbergh, W.C.A.: The Roentgen appearance of ossifying fibroma of bone. Radiology, 50:595-609, 1948.
21. Walker, D.G.: Benign nonodontogenic tumors of the jaws. J. Oral Surg., 28:39-57, 1970.

## CHERUBISM

In 1933, William A. Jones first described familial multilocular cystic disease of the jaws (1). Because the maxillary fullness imparted an upward turning of the eyes, exposing a band of sclera, he assigned the descriptive term "Cherubism" to the disorder.

It was not until 1950 that a patient underwent surgical resection of the jaw and histological examination of the tissue was carried out. The underlying diagnosis of fibrous dysplasia was then established. The cherubic look was explained by the pathological findings of fibrous dysplasia involving the orbit floor and the infraorbital ridge.

There have been few cases reported since the original description more than 45 years ago (1-8). The earliest age of recognition has been 18 months. Cherubism is probably a hereditary disease, transmitted as a dominant with incomplete penetrance in females (2, 3 and 8).

Radiographically, well defined multilocular radiolucent areas, generally equal on both sides of the mandible and maxilla are present (Fig. 48, a, b, c). All areas of the mandible have been involved except the condyles.

Dental abnormalities may be present, the most common of which is the absence of the mandibular second or third molar. On radiographs, displacement of the inferior dental canal and unerupted teeth may be seen. The mandible is always affected, the maxilla less frequently (6). Where the jaws are normal, the teeth are also found to be normal (8). Gradual improvement both clinically and radiographically occur in puberty and continues into adulthood. Regression is seen in girls earlier than in boys (8). In older patients, reports indicate that remodeling occurs with an increase in density and filling in of radiolucent bone (4 and 8).

The striking histopathologic features are a large number of multinucleated giant cells. There is a close resemblance to the reparative giant cell granuloma (5). Between the ages of 20-30, fibrous tissue in the lesion is replaced by sclerotic or normal bone (4).

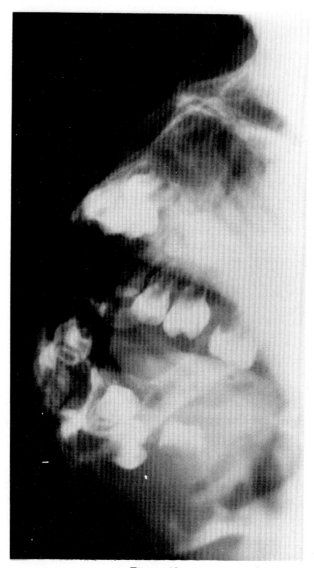

Figure 48a.

Figure 48a-c. Oblique frontal and Waters view in a patient who has familial fibrous dysplasia. These show scalloping and enlargement of the bones of both the mandible and maxilla. (Courtesy of Dr. H. White, Children's Memorial Hospital, Chicago, Illinois.)

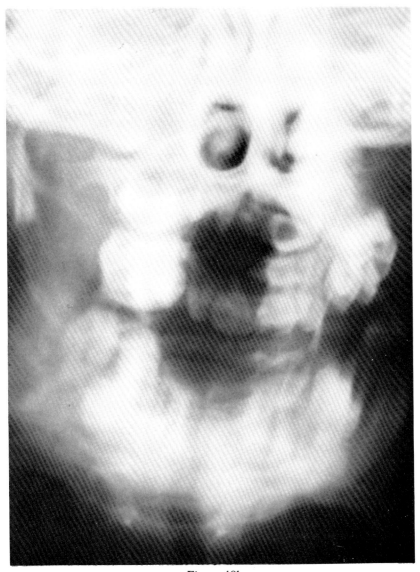

Figure 48b.

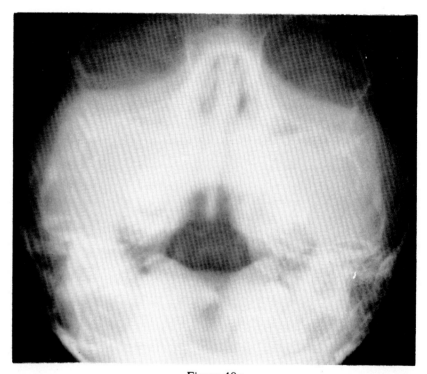

Figure 48c.

## References

1. Jones, W.A.: Familial multilocular cystic disease of the jaws. Am. J. Cancer, 17:946-950, 1933.
2. Anderson, D.E., and McClendon, J.L.: Cherubism: Hereditary fibrous dysplasia of jaws 1. Genetic considerations. Oral Surg., 15 Suppl 2:5-16, 1962.
3. McClendon, J.L., Anderson, D.E., and Cornelius, E.A.: Cherubism: Hereditary fibrous dysplasia of jaws 11. Pathologic considerations. Oral Surg., 15: Suppl 2, 17-42, 1962.
4. Burland, J.E.: Cherubism: Familial bilateral osseous dysplasia of the jaws. Oral Surg., 15: Suppl 2, 43-60, 1962.
5. Hamner, J.E. III: The demonstration of perivascular collagen deposition in cherubism. Oral Surg., 27:129-141, 1969.
6. Cornelius, E.A., and McClendon, J.L.: Cherubism — Hereditary fibrous dysplasia of the jaws. Roentgenographic features. Am. J. Roentgenol., 106:136-143, 1969.
7. Lawrence, D., Nogrady, M.D., and Cloutier, A.M.: Cherubism: A case report. Am. J. Roentgenol., 108:468-472, 1970.
8. Von Wowern, N.: Cherubism. Int. J. Oral Surg., 1:240-249, 1972.

## CEMENTOMA

There are various terms used to described entities that consist of tissue proliferations containing cementum. The most common is periapical cemental (fibrous) dysplasia. On radiographs, it appears early as a well defined radiolucency which later becomes a radiopaque calcified mass (1) (Fig. 49). Initially, this is thought to be the result of a proliferating periodontal ligament which in turn destroys the lamina dura, spreads periapically and replaces bony trabeculae with fibrous connective tissue. The fibrous tissue may then become converted into a calcified mass. The entire process takes from 3-10 years (1 and 3).

It is common in females, in blacks, in persons over 25 years of age and is seen in the mandible. The lesions are often multiple. The gigantiform cementoma (familial multiple cementoma) is densely calcified and may become quite large.

The fibrocementoma is found in the mandible in older individuals and is not associated with teeth. On radiographs, it tends to be mostly radiolucent with some calcified areas.

The benign cementoblastoma occurs at the apex of a tooth, has a rapid rate of growth, is progressive and is sometimes a painful lesion (4 and 5).

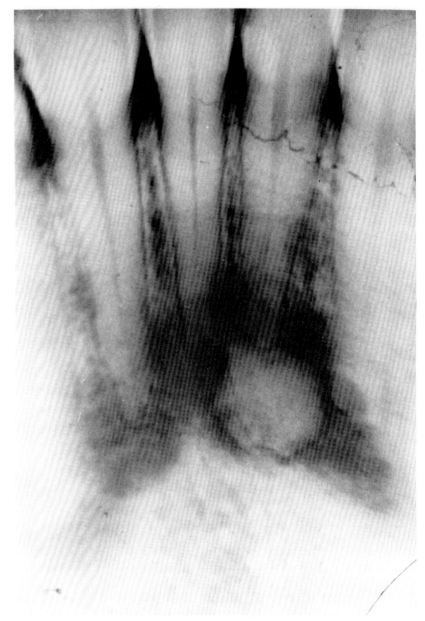

Figure 49. There is a large round density surrounded by an area of radio-lucency at the apex of the roots of the central incisors. This appearance is characteristic of mature periapical fibrous dysplasia (cementoma).

References

1.  Chaudhry, A.P., Spink, J.H., and Gorlin, R.J.: Periapical fibrous dysplasia (cementoma). J. Oral Surg., 16:483-488, 1958.
2.  Waldron, C.A., and Giansanti, J.S.: Benign fibro-osseous lesions of the jaws: A clinical-radiologic-histologic review of sixty-five cases Part II benign fibro-osseous lesion of periodontal ligament origin. Oral Surg., 35:340-350, 1973.
3.  Hamner, J.E., Scofield, H.H., and Cornyn, J.: Benign fibro-osseous jaw lesions of periodontal membrane origin. An analysis of 249 cases. Cancer, 22:861-878, 1968.
4.  Cherrick, H.M., King, O.H., Lucatorto, F.M., and Suggs, D.M.: Benign cementoblastoma. Oral Surg., 37:54-63, 1974.
5.  Larsson, A., Forsberg, O., and Sjorgren, S.: Benign cementoblastomas. J. Oral Surg., 36:299-303, 1978.

# 7

## ACUTE AND CHRONIC OSTEOMYELITIS
## OF THE MANDIBLE

Chronic osteomyelitis of the mandible may follow an acute stage of mandibular osteomyelitis; the acute condition may develop from an infection of dental origin, (Fig. 50 a, b, c) jaw fracture, or a result of extension of local infection in the mouth or nasopharynx (1). Osteomyelitis, as a complication of jaw fractures, is relatively common especially if the bone is not adequately immobilized. Inflammatory changes in the marrow reduce the osteogenic capability of the bone; the periosteum, if involved by the inflammatory process, will also be compressed. Resulting defects may become large enough to require bone grafts (2). Alloplastic implants can represent a nidus for infection since the material is porous (3). Chronic osteomyelitis may also occur after incomplete excision of necrotic bone, or too early termination of antibiotic therapy in patients with jaw infections (Fig. 51). Tuberculous osteomyelitis is a very rare occurrence and appears after the infection arises elsewhere (4), and, when it starts as a periapical infection, in the saliva (5). Tuberculous osteomyelitis as a primary infection although rare has been reported in the area of the maxillary left canine (6).

In chronic osteomyelitis, the infection spreads through the spongiosa, causes a breakdown of the buccal walls of the bone and spreads upwards to the ascending rami, and downwards to the inferior extent of the angles of the mandible. A fistula may be present. On the radiographs, radiolucent areas of destruction of bone, and sequestra may be visible.

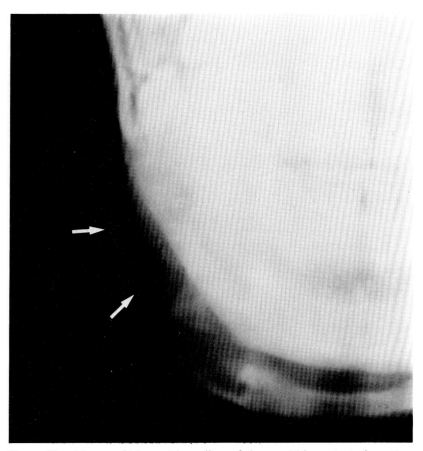

Figure 50a. 10-year-old boy with swelling of the mandible; periosteal reaction is seen on the frontal view *(arrows)*. The bone in this area shows increase in radiolucency.

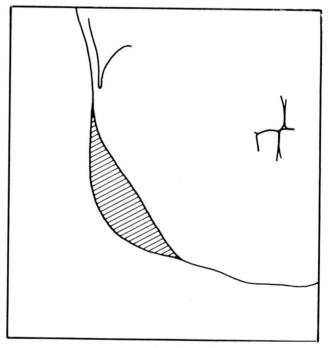

Figure 50b. Sketch.

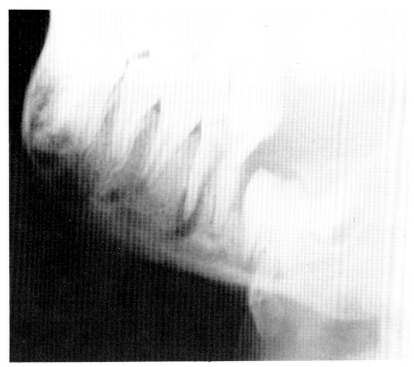

Figure 50c. On the oblique view a carious molar with a periapical abscess is noted to be the source.

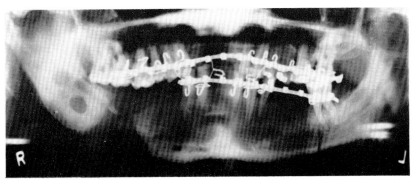

Figure 51. Osteomyelitis at a fracture site with sclerosis of the bone and sequestra.

Sclerosing osteomyelitis represent very chronic forms of inflammation. Local and extensive sclerosing osteomyelitis occurs predominantly in the mandible and appears as radio-opaque areas (Fig. 52 a, b, c). Periosteal new bone is a common feature whereas sequestration is almost never seen (7, 8). On radiographs, osteosclerosis, either poorly defined or with distinct borders is often present (Fig. 52 a, b, c). The sclerotic changes are only present in tooth bearing areas, not the condyles or ascending ramus (8, 10). Tc 99m scintigraphy can be used to determine the extent of the process (10). When extensive, this disorder is called sclerosing osteomyelitis of Garre or condensing osteitis, and is mainly observed in children and young adults. Differentiation from fibrous dysplasia, Ewing's sarcoma and Paget's disease must be made (9, 11).

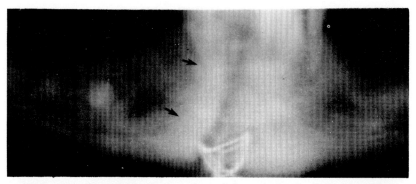

Figure 52a. Cone-down frontal view of the symphysis of the mandible.
Figure 52a-c. Two patients with chronic osteomyelitis showing ill defined areas of osteosclerosis *(arrows)*.

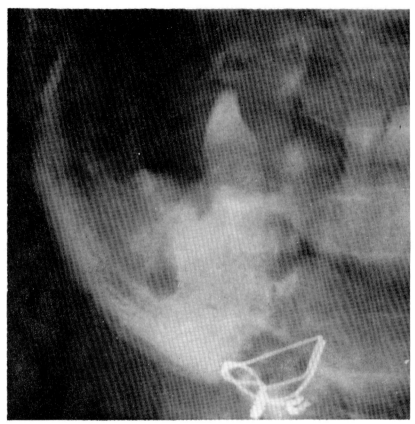

Figure 52b. Oblique view of the area of sclerotic bone.

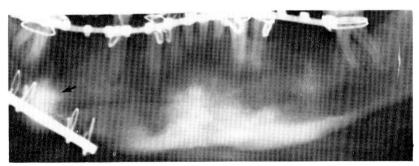

Figure 52c. At the body of the mandible near the metallic plate *(arrow)*.

In osteomyelitis, staphylococci and streptococci are the most common organisms; other organisms such as actinomycosis may be seen (Fig. 53 a, b, c). The actinomycosis fungus is found in the oral flora and enters the bone via a carious tooth, extraction socket or fractured jaw (5).

Osteomyelitis of the newborn is rare and results from infection acquired during delivery. The infant has systemic signs with fever and vomiting. The infection occurs in the maxilla and may develop a draining fistula (12, 14).

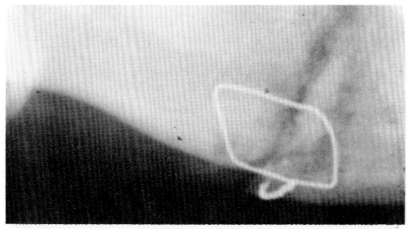

Figure 53a. Cone-down view of the mandible shows poorly healed fracture site.

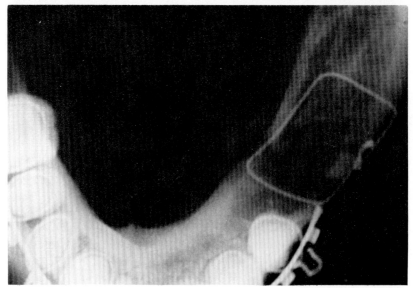

Figure 53b. There is a large area of bony destruction proven to be due to actinomycotic osteomyelitis.

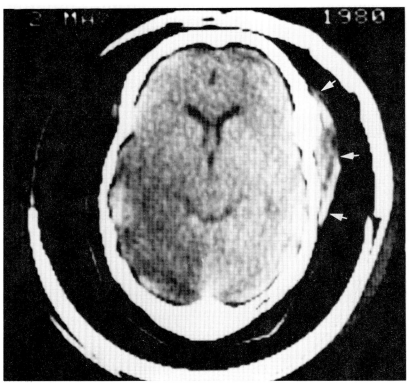

Figure 53c. C.A.T. scan on another patient shows a dense temporalis mass lesion proven pathologically to be due to actinomycosis *(arrows)*.

## References

1. Kinnman, J.E.G., and Lee, H.S.: Chronic osteomyelitis of the mandible: Clinical study of 13 cases. Oral Surg., 25:6-11, 1968.
2. Limongelli, W.A., Connaughton, D., and Williams, A.C.: Suppurative osteomyelitis of the mandible secondary to fracture. Oral Surg., 38:850-859, 1974.
3. Gallagher, D.M., and Epker, B.N.: Infection following intraoral surgical correction of dentofacial deformities: A review of 140 consecutive cases. J. Oral Surg., 38:117-120, 1980.
4. Khosla, V.M.: Tuberculous osteomyelitis of the mandible: Report of case. J. Oral Surg., 28:848-853, 1970.
5. Meyer, I.: Infectious diseases of the jaws. J. Oral Surg., 28:17-28, 1970.
6. Rosenquist, J.B., and Beskow, R.: Tuberculosis of the maxilla: Report of case. J. Oral Surg., 35:309-310, 1977.
7. Wood, N.K., Goaz, P.W., and Stuteville, O.H.: Differential Diagnosis of Oral Lesions. C.V. Mosby 1975. pp. 375-381.
8. Rabe, W.C., Angelillo, J.C., and Leipert, D.W.: Chronic sclerosing osteomyelitis: Treatment considerations in an atypical case. Oral Surg., 49:117-121, 1980.
9. Panders, A.K., and Hadders, H.N.: Chronic sclerosing inflammations of the jaw. Osteomyelitis sicca (Garre). Chronic sclerosing osteomyelitis with fine meshed trabecular structure, and very dense sclerosing osteomyelitis. Oral Surg., 30:396-412, 1970.
10. Jacobsson, S., Hollender, L., Lindberg, S., and Larsson, A.: Chronic sclerosing osteomyelitis of the mandible. Scintigraphic and radiographic findings. Oral Surg., 45:167-174, 1978.
11. Khosla, V.M., Rosenfield, H., and Berk, L.H.: Chronic osteomyelitis of the mandible. J. Oral Surg., 29:649-658, 1971.
12. Hitchin, A.D., and Naylor, M.N.: Acute maxillitis of infancy: Oral Surg., 10:715-724, 1957.
13. Hitchin, A.D., and Naylor, M.N.: Acute maxillitis of infancy: Oral Surg., 18:423-431, 1964.
14. Niego, R.V.: Acute osteomyelitis of the maxilla in the newborn. Oral Surg., 30:611-614, 1970.

# 8

## GENERALIZED DISORDERS
## WITH JAWBONE INVOLVEMENT

### BASAL CELL NEVUS SYNDROME

This syndrome was described as a distinct entity by Gorlin and Goltz in 1960 (1). Previously, there were many scattered reports of basal cell nevus with other anomalies. Straith in 1939 first described jaw cysts in a family with skin lesions (2), Binkley and Johnson in 1951 reported a patient with dental cysts, basal cell nevi, agenesis of the corpus callosum, fibroma of the ovary and bifid ribs (3). Howel and Caro studied anomalies associated with basal cell nevi and mentioned both familial occurrence as well as mandible cysts and multiple skin cancers (4). The syndrome is less common among blacks although several families have been reported (5, 6).

Synonyms for this syndrome include multiple basal cell nevi syndrome, nevoid, basal cell carcinoma syndrome. To complete the syndrome, multiple basal cell nevi (Fig. 54), jaw cysts (Fig. 55) and skeletal anomalies are invariably present, but there are other clinical features such as unusual facies due to frontal and temporoparietal bossing, pronounced supraorbital ridges, broad nasal root, large superciliar ridge marking and eyes appearing wide and deep (7, 12).

There have been multiple reports of other defects in the syndrome including short fourth metacarpal, dyskeratosis of the palms and soles, calcification in the falx cerebri, meningioma, medulloblastoma, scoliosis, skin cysts, prognathism, mental retardation and hyporesponsiveness to parathyroid horomone (11, 13).

The jaw cysts are most often multilocular keratocysts which recur frequently, and usually appear in childhood or early adulthood. In many reported cases the primary complaint has been due to swelling, and displacement of teeth. Secondary infection may produce pain and drainage (10). In contrast to solitary keratocysts, the distribution is not isolated to the angle and ramus of the mandible (7), although in most patients with the syndrome multiple radiolucencies in either jaw close to the teeth may appear (10). On radiographs, the cysts have a scalloped outline, sometimes multilocular (7) and may contain unerupted displaced teeth (Fig. 2). Cysts appear before the expected eruption dates in Rayne's series (15). Multiplicity, bilaterality and continuous development of the jaw cysts were present in a family described by Anderson (16).

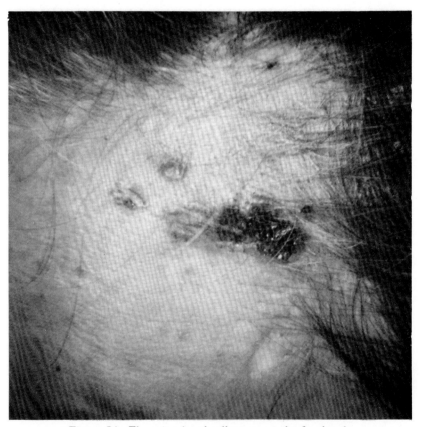

Figure 54. There is a basal cell nevus on the forehead.

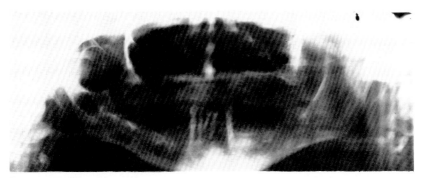

Figure 55. Panorex demonstrates multiple cysts in the body and ramus of the right mandible associated with basal cell nevus syndrome.

## References

1. Gorlin, R.J., and Goltz, R.W.: Multiple nevoid basal-cell epithelioma, jaw cysts and bifid rib: A syndrome. NEJM, 262:908-912, 1960.
2. Straith, F.E.: Hereditary epidermoid cyst of the jaws. Am. J. Orthod. and Oral Surg., 25:637, 1939.
3. Binkley, G.W., and Johnson, H.H.: Epithelioma adenoides cysticum: Basal cell nevi, agenesis of the corpus callosum and dental cysts. AMA Arch Derm., 63:78-84, 1951.
4. Howell, J.B., and Caro, M.R.: The basal-cell nevus. Its relationship to multiple cutaneous cancers and associated anomalies of development. AMA Arch Derm., 79:67-80, 1959.
5. Giansanti, J.S., and Baker, G.O.: Nevoid basal cell carcinoma syndrome in negroes: Report of five cases. J. Oral Surg., 32:138-144, 1974.
6. Ryan, D.E., and Burkes, E.J.: The multiple basal-cell nevus syndrome in a negro family. Oral Surg., 36:831-835, 1973.
7. Donatsky, O., Hjörting-Hansen, E., Philipsen, H.P., and Fejerskov, O.: Clinical radiologic and histopathologic aspects of 13 cases of nevoid basal cell carcinoma syndrome. Int. J. Oral Surg., 5:19-28, 1976.
8. Koutnick, A.W., Kolodny, S.C., Hooker, S.P., and Roche, W.C.: Multiple nevoid basal cell epithelioma, cysts of the jaw, and bifid rib syndrome: Report of case. J. Oral Surg., 33:606-669, 1975.
9. Schwartz, S.H., Blankenship, B.J., and Stout, R.A.: Multiple basal cell nevus syndrome: Report of case. J. Oral Surg., 28:523-527, 1970.
10. Berlin, N.I., Van Scott, E.J., Clendenning, W.E., Archard, H.O., Block, J.B., Witkop, C.J., and Haynes, H.A.: Basal cell nevus syndrome. Combined clinical staff conference at the national institutes of health. Ann. Intern. Med., 64:403-421, 1966.

11. Gilhuus-Moe, O., Haugen, L.K., and Dee, P.M.: The syndrome of multiple cysts of the jaws, basal cell carcinomata and skeletal anomalies. Br. J. Oral Surg., 5:211-222, 1968.

12. Rater, C.J., Selke, A.C., and Van Epps, E.F.: Basal cell nevus syndrome. Amer. J. Roentgol., 103:589-594, 1968.

13. Stoelinga, P.J.W., Peters, J.H., van de Staak, W.J., and Cohen, M.W.: Some new findings in the basal-cell nevus syndrome. Oral Surg., 36:686-692, 1973.

14. Gorlin, R.J., Vickers, R.A., Kellin, E., and Williamson, J.J.: The multiple basal-cell nevi syndrome. An analysis of a syndrome consisting of multiple nevoid basal-cell carcinoma, jaw cysts, skeletal anomalies, medulloblastoma, and hyporesponsiveness to parathormone. Cancer, 18:89-104, 1965.

15. Rayne, J.: The multiple basal cell naevi syndrome. Br. J. Oral Surg., 9:65-71, 1971.

16. Anderson, D.E., and Cook, W.A.: Jaw cysts and the basal cell nevus syndrome. J. Oral Surg., 24:15-26, 1966.

## GARDNER'S SYNDROME

Gardner's syndrome is an inherited disorder with a characteristic triad of defects including colon polyps, osteomas and soft tissue tumors. Dental anomalies are common and seen early in the disease, frequently before other manifestations. In Gardner and Stenves original reports, all nine patients had osteomas of the mandible or calvarium (1, 2). It is now known that external manifestations precede gastrointestinal disease; the appearance of osteomas and dental anomalies may alert the clinician to have patients endoscoped and examined for polyps and other gastrointestinal tumors (3). Even if the family history is inconclusive, colonic malignancy may appear (4).

Osteomas of the jaw appear in young patients. The mandible is more commonly involved showing areas of increased density and protuberant osteoma (Fig. 56 a, b, c). These tumors are also found in the maxilla and other facial bones (Fig. 57). They may appear in long bones as irregular cortical elevations or osteomas. In the mandible, the osteomas are attached to the external cortex of the body and ramus (5, 7). Growing bone lesions appearing as fibrous dysplasia on radiographs have been reported (8).

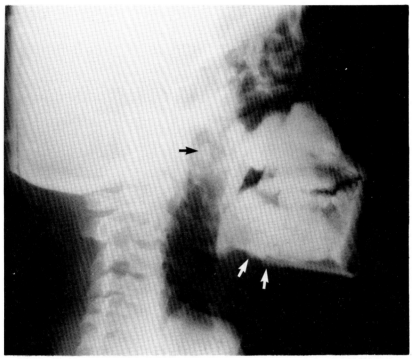

Figure 56a. A 15-year-old boy presented with osteomas of the mandible *(arrows)*.

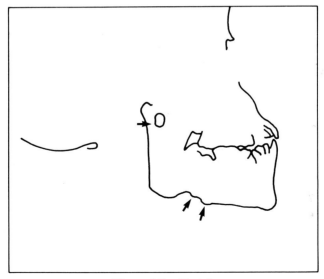

Figure 56b. Sketch.

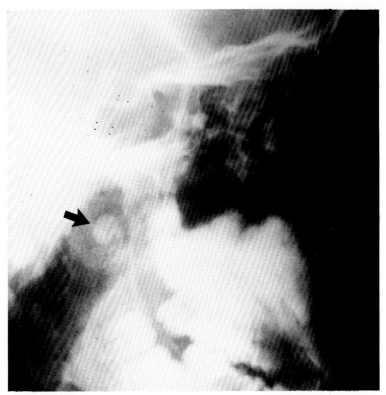

Figure 56c. Additional osteomata were found on the lateral view of the face *(arrow)*.

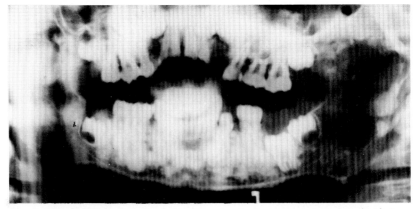

Figure 57. Multiple impacted teeth and odontomata are seen in both jaws in a patient with Gardner's syndrome.

Dental abnormalities including carious teeth, loss of normal trabecular pattern, unerupted and supernumerary teeth have been observed as features of the syndrome (5, 9) (Fig. 3). These impacted teeth were composed of normal dental structures and were of various size and shape. There is speculation that these may represent denticles in compound odontomata (10) (Fig. 58).

Maxilla or mandible may show replacement of bony trabeculae by irregular, dense bone (5, 6). Other malignancies have been reported in the syndrome: osteogenic sarcoma (9), chondrosarcoma of the hyoid bone (11).

Desmoid tumors have been noted as part of the syndrome. These tumors arise from connective tissue, in fascia and muscle, and commonly occur in the anterior abdominal wall, are locally infiltrative and may grow to a great size but rarely metastasize (12).

The polyposis in Gardner's syndrome develops in childhood or adult life and are usually multiple (6). The malignant potential is high and malignant degeneration of intestinal polyps is an inevitable development (12). The disorder is inherited as an autosomal dominant (2, 6, 12).

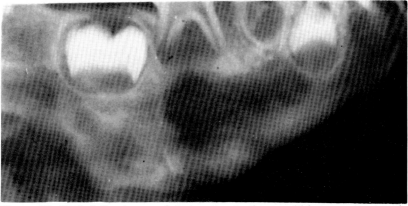

Figure 58. Well defined area of destruction in the mandible in a patient with Hand-Schuller Christian disease.

## References

1. Gardner, E.J., and Richards, R.C.: Multiple cutaneous and subcutaneous lesions occurring simultaneously with hereditary polyposis and osteomatosis. Am. J. Hum. Genet., 5:137-139, 1953.
2. Gardner, E.J.: Follow-up study of a Family Group Exhibiting Dominant Inheritance for a Syndrome Including Intestinal Polyps, Osteomas, Fibromas and Eipdermal cysts. Am. J. Hum. Genet., 14:376-390, 1962.
3. Sanchez, M.A., Zali, M.R., Khalil, A.A., Ponce, R., and Font, R.G.: Be aware of Gardner's syndrome. Am. J. Gastroenterol., 71:68-73, 1979.
4. Halse, A., Roed-Petersen, B., and Lund, K.: Gardner's syndrome. J. Oral Surg., 33:673-675, 1975.
5. Fader, M., Kline, S.N., Spatz, S.S., and Zubrow, H.J.: Gardner's syndrome (intestinal polyposis, osteomas, sebaceous cysts) and a new dental discovery. Oral Surg., 15:153-172, 1962.
6. Jones, E.L., and Cornell, W.P.: Gardner's syndrome. Review of the literature and report on a family. Arch. Surg., 92:287-300, 1966.
7. Amato, A.E., and Small, E.W.: Oral manifestations of Gardner's syndrome: Report of case. J. Oral Surg., 28:458-460, 1970.
8. Small, I.P., Shandler, H., Husain, M., and David, H.: Gardner's syndrome with an unusual fibro-osseous lesion of the mandible. Oral Surg., 49:477-485, 1980.
9. Chang, C.H., Piatt, E.D., Thomas, K.E., and Watne, A.L.: Bone abnormalities in Gardner's syndrome. Amer. J. Roentgenol., 103:645-652, 1968.
10. Davies, A.S.: Gardner's syndrome: A case report. Br. J. Oral Surg., 51-57, 1969.
11. Greer, J.A., Devine, K.D., and Dahlin, D.C.: Gardner's syndrome and chondrosarcoma of the hyoid bone. Arch. Otolaryngol., 103:425-427, 1977.
12. Santos, M.J., Krush, A.J., and Cameron, J.L.: Three varieties of hereditary intestinal polyposis. The Johns Hopkins Medical Journal, 145:196-200, 1979.

## HISTIOCYSTOSIS X

Histiocystosis X is the term for a complex group of diseases of the reticuloendothelial system. The acute form seen in infants is called Letterer-Siwe Disease, the chronic form Hand-Schuller-Christian disease. Solitary lesions are considered eosinophilic granulomas.

Letterer-Siwe disease, which occurs in infants and children almost always younger than three years, has a rampant course with the appearance of many skin lesions including papulopustular exanthema, petichiae and seborrheic dermatitis (1, 2). Bone defects are usually extensive. Hand-Schuller-Christian disease occurs predominantly in older children and young adults in a male-female ratio of 3 to 2.

In Hand-Schuller-Christian disease, granulomas develop in flatbones, especially in the skull or mandible (Figs. 58, 59). These lesions may progress rapidly and according to the location of the pathologic process, give rise to symptoms. Exophthalmos develops when the orbital wall is involved, diabetes insipidus results when the sella turcica and pituitary are destroyed.

On radiographs, eosinophilic granuloma of bone presents as a benign well localized radiolucent lesion round, oval or irregular with cortical erosion on the medullary side and sometimes cortical thickening on the periosteal side (3, 5, 6). A thin zone of sclerosis may surround the osteolytic lesion. Pathological fractures and periosteal new bone may appear. On occasions, there may be difficulty in classifying the three separate entities and possibly there may be progression from one to another more extensive disease (4).

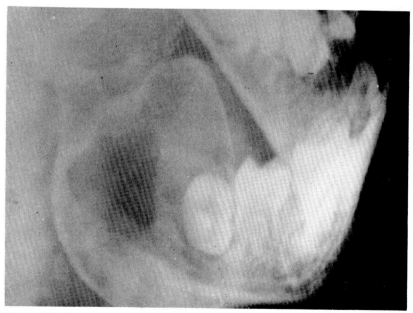

Figure 59. Destructive radiolucent lesion in the ramus of the mandible extending into the condyle in a case of Hand-Schuller-Christian disease. (Courtesy of Dr. H. White, Children's Memorial Hospital, Chicago, Illinois.)

In the jaw, the mandible is most frequently involved (7). Oral manifestations may represent early findings in the disease, and sore mouth, loose and sore teeth, pain and swelling may be some of the findings (8, 9). In children, eruption and looseness of permanent teeth, advanced periodontal disease, and failure of a socket to heal after a tender loose tooth is extracted are signs of the disease (8, 11). The radiographic appearances varies depending on the presence of teeth.

Floating teeth (Figs. 60-61) appear when resorption of an alveolar bone occurs. However, radiographic findings may not be specific and may resemble periapical or cystic lesions. The radiographic appearance may be that of sharp well circumscribed radiolucent areas (3, 7, 11), although margins of the lesions vary from well defined to indistinct (Fig. 62). Initial involvement may be in the molar and premolar regions where destruction of the alveolar bone is seen. Anterior parts of the jaw are involved later in the course of the disease. Pathological fractures of the mandible are not common (8). Involvement of the jaw by isolated eosinophilic granuloma is uncommon and biopsy is required to confirm the diagnosis.

$\longrightarrow$

Figure 61. Close up view of "Floating teeth" in a child with eosinophilic granuloma.

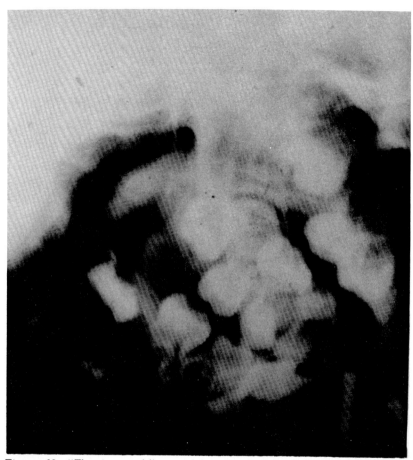

Figure 60. "Floating teeth" caused by destruction of alveolar bone of the mandible.

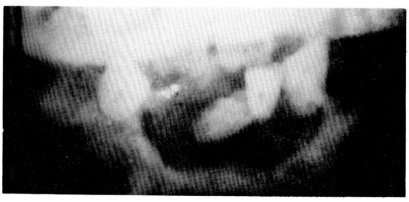

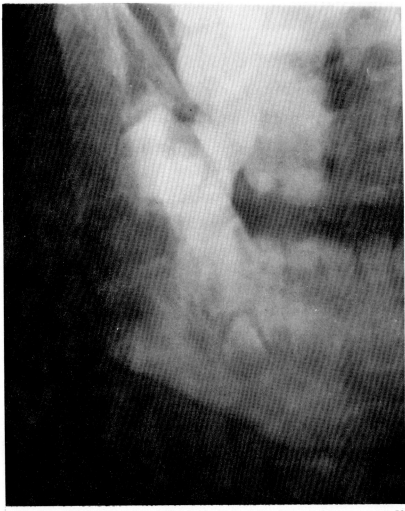

Figure 62. Expansion and destruction of the mandible in histiocystosis X. (Courtesy of Dr. H. White, Children's Memorial Hospital, Chicago, Illinois.)

References

1. Dargeon, H.W.: Considerations in the treatment of reticuloendotheliosis. Am. J. Roentgenol., 93:521-536, 1965.
2. Nyholm, K.: Eosinophilic xanthomatous granulomatosis and Letterer-Siwe's disease. Acta. Pathol. Microbiol. Scand., 1971 A. Suppl, 216.
3. Sleeper, E.L.: Eosinophilic granuloma of bone. Its relationship to Hand-Schuller-Christian and Letterer-Siwe's diseases, with emphasis upon oral symptoms and findings. Oral Surg., 4:896-918, 1951.
4. Snyder, S.R., Merkow, L.P., and White, N.S.: Eosinophilic granuloma of bone: Report of case. J. Oral Surg., 31:712-715, 1973.
5. Dundon, C.C., Williams, H.A., and Laipply, T.C.: Eosinophilic granuloma of bone. Radiology, 47:433-444, 1946.
6. Hamilton, J.B., Barner, J.L., Kennedy, P.C., and McCort, J.J.: Osseous manifestations of eosinophilic granuloma: Report of nine cases. Radiology, 47:445-456, 1946.
7. Jones, J.C., Lilly, G.E., and Marlette, R.H.: Histiocystosis X. J. Oral Surg., 28:461-469, 1970.
8. Blevins, C., Dahlin, D.C., Lovestedt, S.A., and Kennedy, R.L.J.: Oral and Dental manifestations of histiocystosis X. Oral Surg., 12:473-483, 1959.
9. Scott, J., and Finch, L.D.: Histiocystosis X with oral lesions: Report of case. J. Oral Surg., 30:748-753, 1972.
10. Whitehead, F.I.H.: Histiocystosis X. Brit. J. Oral Surg., 10:199-204, 1972.
11. Shklar, G., Taylor, R., and Schwartz, S.: Oral lesions of eosinophilic granuloma. Oral Surg., 19:613-622, 1965.

## INFANTILE CORTICAL HYPEROSTOSIS

Infantile cortical hyperostosis (Caffey's disease) affects infants under the age of five months. There is a sudden onset of soft tissue swelling of the face or extremities, irritability and x-ray appearance of cortical or periosteal new bone. In the majority of patients, the disease is self limited and the bony changes disappear within one year. Almost invariably, the mandible is affected (1) (Fig. 63 a, b, c, d). Children studied for dental defects 1 3/4 or 6 11/12 years after the initial episode had mild residual deformities, cortical thickening or slight mandibular asymmetry. The teeth including enamel and eruptive sequence were normal (2).

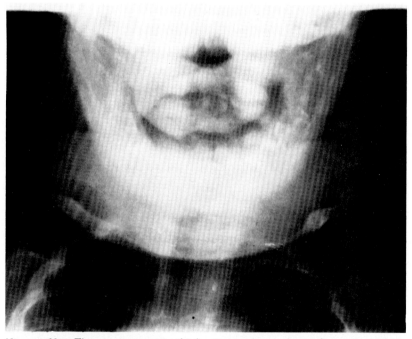

Figure 63a. There is extensive thickening and new bone formation of the entire mandible in a 4-month-old male.

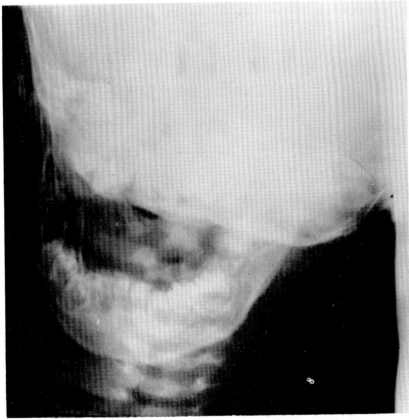

Figure 63b. Healing of the mandible four (4) months later.

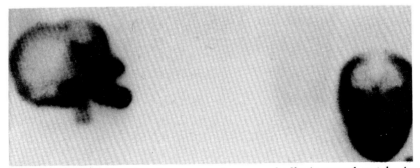

Figure 63c. A Technetium bone scan shows markedly increased uptake in the region of the mandible.

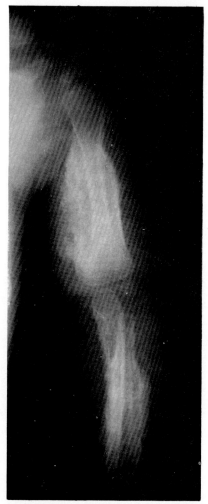

Figure 63d. There is extensive periosteal new bone along the shafts of the left humerus, radius and ulna.

## References

1.  Caffey, John: Infantile cortical Hyperostosis. J. Pediatr., 29:541-559, 1946.
2.  Burband, P.M., Lovestedt, S.A., Kennedy, R.L.J.: The dental aspect of infantile cortical hyperostosis. Oral Surg., 11:1126-1137, 1958.

# AUTHOR INDEX

## A

Abrams, A.M., 39, 40, 64
Adekeye, E.O., 59
Ajaqbe, H.A., 42
Alford, B.A., 116
Allen, J.W., 39, 51
Allen, P.M., 77
Amato, A.E., 156
Anderson, D.E., 137, 150, 152
Angelillo, J.C., 148
Archard, H.O., 151
Ariel, I.M., 81
Austine, L.T., 39

## B

Baden, E., 39
Bahn, S.L., 40
Baker, C.G., 106
Baker, G.O., 151
Barber, T.K., 93
Barner, J.L., 161
Barnfield, W.F., 60
Barry, R.J., 132
Batsakis, J.G., 81
Becker, R., 51
Berger, A., 132
Berlin, N.I., 151
Berk, L.H., 148
Bernier, J.L., 42, 51, 93
Beskow, R., 148
Besse, B.E., 51
Bhasker, S.N., 40, 51, 60, 64
Biehl, D.L., 39
Biesecker, J.L., 51
Binkley, G.W., 149, 151
Birn, H., 40, 64
Blankenship, B.J., 151
Blevins, C., 161
Block, J.B., 151

Block, J.C., 93
Bolden, T.E., 77
Borello, E.D., 93
Brekke, J.H., 93
Bruce, K.W., 77
Brueggemann, A., 4
Bullock, W.K., 39, 51
Burband, P.M., 164
Burkes, E.J., 151
Burkitt, D., 106, 107, 108, 110, 112,
114, 116
Burland, J.E., 137
Byrd, D.L., 39, 51

## C

Caffey, J., 164
Cameron, J.L., 156
Campbell, J.J., 39
Cangiano, R., 132
Caro, R.F., 60
Caruso, W., 77
Castner, E.V., 52, 59
Chambers, K.S., 64
Chang, C.H., 156
Chaudry, A.P., 64, 139
Cherrick, H.M., 139
Christiansen, G.W., 106, 116
Church, L.E., 132
Ciola, B., 40
Clendenning, W.E., 151
Clough, J.R., 51
Cloutier, A.M., 137
Cocci, P.R., 116
Cockshott, W.P., v, 107, 108, 110,
112, 114, 116
Cohen, M.W., 152
Connaughton, D., 148
Cook, W.A., 152
Cornelius, E.A., 137
Cornell, W.P., 156

165

# SUBJECT INDEX

## A

Actinomycosis,
  origin of, 146
  temporalis lesion, Fig. 53c, 147
Adeno-ameloblastoma,
  and dentigerous cysts,
    differentiation, 60
  frequent site, 60
  occurrence frequency, 60
  odontogenic origin,
    and embedded tooth, 60, 61, 62,
    63
  Water's view, 23a, 61
Albright's syndrome,
  lesion association, 117, 124
Ameloblastic adenomatoid tumor. *See
  also* Tumors.
Ameloblastic fibroma. *See also*
  Odontoma
Ameloblastic odontoma. *See also*
  Odontoma
Ameloblastoma,
  and follicular cysts, 52
  appearance on radiographs, 58
  as unilocular cavity,
    Fig. 22a showing, 58
  composition of, 52
  differential diagnosis, 58
  malignant potential, 52
  maxilla involvement, 52
  metastases to lungs, 58
  name origin, 52
  radiographic appearance, 58
  radiographs, 53, 54, 55, 56, 57

## B

Bone,
  alveolar,
    destruction, Fig. 60, 159

aneurysmal, 42-43
eosinophilic granuloma, 157
grafts needed,
  in osteomyelitis, 140
humerus, radius, ulna,
  Fig. 63d, 164
in fibrous dysplasia, 120, 121
in sarcoma, 94, 106-110
membranous,
  ossifying fibroma in, 128
necrotic,
  osteomyelitis resulting, 140
with fibrous dysplasia, 124

## C

Caffey's disease. *See also* Hyperostosis.
Carcinoma,
  basal cell syndrome., 149
  squamous cell,
    axial C. T. scans, 104, 105
    clinical findings, 100
    erosive, Fig. 36a, 102
    jaw size increase, 100
    mandible expansion, 102
    median age for, 100
    origin of, 28, 100
    ulceration, Fig. 36c, 103
Cementoma,
  periapical dysplasia, 137-138
Cherubism. *See also* Dysplasia.
Chondrosarcoma. *See also* Sarcoma.
Cysts,
  aneurysmal bone,
    ameloblastoma, 43
    bone replacement, 43
    etiology, 42-43
    fistulas, 43
    histological examination, 43, 47
    occurrence of, 42
    radiograph results, 43, 44, 46, 47

V

W

X

Y

U